SONIA MARIE TRIMBLE

Little Miss Healthy Pants

Fit Happens

A Novel

Sonia Marie Trimble
5953 West Park Avenue
Houma, Louisiana/70364
www.littlemisshealthypants.com

Publisher's Note: This is a work of fiction. Names, characters, places, and incidents are a product of the author's imagination. Locales and public names are sometimes used for atmospheric purposes. Any resemblance to actual people, living or dead, or to businesses, companies, events, institutions, or locales is completely coincidental.

Book Cover Design & Layout ©2015 Createspace.com
Chapter Illustrations ©2014 JesseBibbs.com

Ordering Information:
Quantity sales. Special discounts are available on quantity purchases by corporations, associations, and others. For details, contact the "Special Sales Department" at the address above.

Little Miss Healthy Pants Fit Happens/
Sonia Marie Trimble. -- 1st ed.
ISBN 978-1507573327

Contributed to those who fight to balance the hilarity and hard work of dealing with both sides of being your own best friend and absolute worst enemy through the choices and challenges of making fit and healthy a lifestyle.

Introduction

When I began penning the idea of Little Miss Healthy Pants on a scrap sheet of paper, which I've sentimentally kept for testimony of what a random doodle session can ultimately create, I knew I didn't want to convey the story of our main character, Whitney Cordona, as a simple narrative of "She lost weight, and now she feels great!" It's rarely that simple.

Throughout my seven years and counting of laboring to help people of various fitness backgrounds and physiques cultivate a fit and healthy lifestyle, I've grown to understand how often the choices and challenges in one's personal fitness journey can take that individual through total highs and terrible lows, all in the same day. And while I've connected with most everyone from teens to adults and apprentices to athletes in my career, Whitney's story, and each individual and detail that surrounds it, is purely a work of fiction. Furthermore, the insight and fitness tips discussed in this fictional story are not recommended to be utilized outside of the instruction and/or directives of one's physician.

With Fit Happens being my first novel, it was slightly exhilarating yet unbelievably distressing to pen the details of Whitney's story in her own entertaining yet often impolite voice. She reveals her pains and disappointments in manners that may offend us a bit while it reminds us that neither of us, nor our journey, is a typical version of anyone or anything. Whether we're one of hundreds on a bustling gym floor or one of dozens in an electrifying fitness class, our personal fitness journey is like no other, although the experiences of others can personally impact and inspire our efforts.

What's more, with the audacity of a wet behind the ears author, I portrayed Whitney as both the villain and the heroine of her own thought-provoking story. Nonetheless, I trust that you, the reader, will appreciate the fact that not a single person will love or loathe Whitney, nor help or harm her, nearly as much as she'll personally determine to do so throughout her every choice and challenge. Just as we must choose to courageously recognize in our own personal lives, her plight confirms the truth that no one has the ultimate capability to rescue our life, or ruin it, outside of our own decisions and determinations.

From the challenges in both her family and career relationships, to the life transforming experience with a personal trainer that will not only bring her to the mountaintop of accomplishment in her goals but

*also to the valley of contemplating total defeat yet
again, Whitney's rollercoaster tale is filled with raw
emotion as it reminds us that every worthwhile
journey bears difficulty as we push forward to bring
forth the champion on the inside of us.*

*May Whitney's story offer us complete hope and
further clarity of what can happen when Fit Happens.*

CHAPTER ONE

Big Girls Don't Cry; We Bite

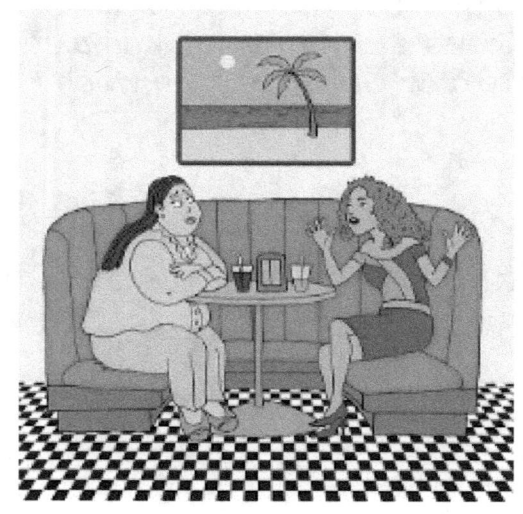

"Ok, great! So, that's two orders of the steak fajita plate with extra sour cream and extra guacamole with each. I'll have those entrees out shortly for you ladies," our waiflike waitress responded with what I'm sure was a smirk as she gathered up the menus while assuming she'd completed our entire order.

"No, I ordered both of those entrees for myself. My cousin will be ordering for herself," I responded with an annoyance I didn't care to hide anymore. "It's our cheat day, and I'm going to enjoy two of your practically miniature sized fajita plates. So, I'd rather you give the same odd look you gave when I ordered dessert first instead of the way you're gawking at me now. As if I've ordered the entire kitchen when you and I know this restaurant is one of the only in Dallas where almost every entrée consists of children's sized portions."

Although Barb and I loved the flavors and festive atmosphere of Rocko's Caribbean Grill, I often felt we paid more for the party atmosphere than the obviously rationed portions of the entrées. It took more effort to stuff our faces to satisfaction from the menu than it took to shove myself into a form fitting dress during a good week on my bathroom scale.

"I do apologize ma'am. I didn't mean to offend you. I assumed the order you gave was for both of you ladies," she replied with a smile which didn't hide her undoubtedly chastened expression.

"Well, bless your lean little heart. Haven't you heard what happens when we assume things? It makes an ass out of you and me. As you've clearly seen, I'm sitting on way too big of an ass to add anymore to the ambience at our table," I snickered at her, longing for her lanky frame to disappear from our table as soon as possible. All I wanted was to eat heartily and not be reminded of what I could possibly look like if I chose to eat much of nothing as she apparently did. The fact I'd sensed her judgment of me from the moment she came to our table and concluded I was clearly the one who wouldn't be leaving anything on my plate left me even more annoyed than the wait I knew we'd have to endure to receive our food.

"Our apologies. My usually charming cousin is just having a tough week as you may be too," Barb smiled at the ethereal waitress in a repentant voice, attempting to assure she was okay. "I'll have the fajita plate also, with chicken and no sour cream. Thank you."

"Thank you. I'll get those out to you ladies without delay," she smiled faintly at Barb, avoiding any further eye contact with me before scurrying away with our orders.

"Tough week or not, I won't be judged for eating whatever I want on my cheat day," I looked directly at Barb with my *don't even try to defend her* face as the willowy waitress faded from our view. "I didn't mean to be so harsh to her, but it's a new year. I won't tolerate the same old demeaning looks from anyone like her. I could feel her sneers at me from the moment she came prancing to our table with those terrific legs as her terrific hair tossed about too terrifically on her terrific little frame. Her entire persona screams she has no idea what it's like to look forward to eating. And, I'm sure she won't harm our meals, Barb. It appears she's fashioned an allergy to food." I finished with my heated hilarity. I felt no remorse in giving our picture-perfect waitress a dose of the disdain I absorbed daily.

"You don't know her story, Whit, although it's terrifically detailed in your head." Barb chuckled apprehensively, staring a bit blankly at my sinister smile. "I don't think the young lady meant any harm.

You can't continue going around thinking everyone is judging you, and then being so combative about it even if it may be the case. You've represented such a well-known and now overly publicized med spa in this city. All Dallas needs is one more despicable professional who's known for not being pleasant or professional at all," she scolded with a faint smile.

Barb's point was duly noted, I thought momentarily about the current details of my life and career being in utter flux. My life was fairly comfy as a Physician Assistant in Dermatology despite my existing job status of having to abruptly replace my dream job in a city I totally loved within a body I oftentimes hated. The splendor of Dallas' substantial skyline and plethora of prominent communities was the perfect backdrop for the lifestyle I cultivated alongside Barb, her family, and all of our connecting family and friends. Dallas' long hot summers caused us to crave for the brief winter season, until a randomly snow filled winter triggered our yearning for the signature hot temperatures again. We'd grown to embrace the inconsistent weather surrounding a mostly consistent Southern charm in a fashion forward city flanked with countless upscale settings of fun and festivities. While it infuriated me that my heavy frame was limited in relishing the limitless trendy shopping options encircling the township where we resided in North Dallas, I certainly enjoyed the mouthwatering cuisines pouring out from innovative restaurants and diverse eateries which sprang up more often than the yellow daffodils in the city's brief spring season.

11

Nevertheless, I had to agree with Barb. I had no capacity for another public disgrace or catastrophe to be placed on my personal list of life challenges.

"Maybe you're right. But, more importantly, thank you for choosing the best place on our top ten list we indulge on our cheat day," I chortled, returning to devouring the mouth-watering turtle a la mode cheesecake while intentionally changing the subject from Barb's annoying advice and futile attempt to make me play nice in public. She and I were aware of the continuous twice over looks I received whenever I was out with her, being twice her size in every facet of my body. I was done playing nice or fair amongst individuals who had no desire to do so in regards to fatties like me.

"Yeah, I still love it here too. It's the least I can do since this hasn't been the best week for either of us," she responded without her standard sunburst smile.

"Yeah, we've seen much better days," I agreed, taking another huge bite for comfort.

Although I knew my pants would pay the price later, I was depending on every morsel of the gourmet cheesecake I was gobbling to settle at least a few of the annoyances of the hour as we awaited our entrées. Even so, Barb was right. Our current reality was reality. There I was again, all set and reluctantly ready to go for another life induced do-over, as if I hadn't already spent the past few years desperately attempting to stand strong on my big fat feet. I tried my damnedest not to complain, but after already surviving the classic humiliating divorce, leaving me and my then 8-year-old Emily emotionally destitute, I wasn't looking forward to another life-sized challenge to my strength or my sanity.

If I had to hear my expensive therapist declare once again that I'm so capable of getting through most any circumstance if I'm but willing to do the work, I'd go into a screaming ft on her vintage leather couch. I'd leave her wishing she filled our time with far more than her nauseatingly positive clichés. Then again, if it weren't for my time with Dr. Lansing, my ex, Julian, would've a ready been found near dead amongst a few dumbbells—dumbbells which were unquestionably named for his obnoxiously gorgeous workout buddy girlfriend who grasped much of nothing in life outside of fashion and how to maintain her twiggy frame required to prance around in the couture threads she paraded outside the gym.

Julian had been a fairly patient and understanding husband at first, as I made every effort to shed the numerous pounds I'd steadily gained before and after Emily's arrival. Throughout our twelve years of marriage he seriously maintained our early on pact to stay in shape no matter what, continuing to workout solo, keeping his 6'1" brown-eyed, dark-haired frame chiseled with every muscle I always melted over.

Though I initially fought hard to get back on course with him, defeat after defeat in my weight loss goals eventually led me to fight his exhausting efforts to help, fiercely reminding him my choices

13

concerning my health and fitness were ultimately *my* choices. Yet, this did nothing to stop him in pursuing his passion to see a transformation of my increasingly heavy frame, consistently making healthy choices for us whether we ate in or ate out, pleading with me to get my mojo back. He yearned for me to rediscover the eager workout buddy and enthusiastic lover he so desperately missed. At least that's how he explained it at first.

As his concerned persistence grew into irritating jabs, and my promises of continued effort changed to proud defiance, we did what I am sure most exhausted couples often choose to do. We blamed. We threatened. And, we ultimately ignored. We blatantly disregarded each other and solidified the fact we no longer had any real connection or desire to interact beyond parenting Emily, which was mostly done solo as we subtly began to split family time in order to avoid constant confrontations and increasingly phony conversations. And, in a conclusion more dramatic than the countless arguments that preceded it, we officially and completely fell apart when Julian could no longer ignore his longing to find comfort in a more captivating and compliant someone else.

On many occasions in therapy, I chuckled at the memory of my charging the pair of them with the waffle maker. I hoped to smash their cheating faces into that stainless grid iron on what was the worst day of my life as a woman: the day I walked into my home to find my husband locked with another woman in a kiss more passionate than he and I had shared in ages. My heart shattered and my mind fell apart as I beheld him groping her body in hunger, apparently because my hunger for all things food had expanded my frame far beyond a physique he desired to grope or even touch anymore.

After a few years and ever more tears, I learned to decide it was fantastically fantastic when Emily returned home after another fun visit with Daddy announcing news about him and Karen: news about how they'd redesigned the sunroom into an awesome home gym. I was offersively thrilled that they'd fashioned a habitation where they could continue to enjoy their every moment of sweating profusely through sets of silly exercises and slurping smoothies.

The betrayal of their affair wounded my heart more than the shame scarred my soul. Karen was a childhood friend whom no one would've imagined to become my most hated enemy as she became my husband's chosen lover. When we'd all welcomed her back into the fold upon her return to Dallas after her horrific divorce in New York City, I would've never predicted the welcome mat would lead her fit and foul physique directly to our bedroom. Especially considering upon her arrival, she immediately began dating our mutual friend, Ian.

Ian was a charming blond haired, 6-foot frame of sincere smiles and a solid physique who had also withstood an awful public divorce, and Karen was no doubt everything that most any available man would want. She flaunted an hourglass figure which hadn't been weathered by the tough process of childbearing or the stress of any challenging job beyond fighting the Barney's Christmas crowd in New York City where she'd been a well-kept woman in her 15-year marriage: a marriage that crashed as colossally as an exquisite vase in the midst of an exclusive dinner party when her ex-husband disposed of her in order to move on. Get this, with the fresh out of college realtor who had assisted in the purchase of their posh Manhattan apartment. Had I known the treachery of Karen's soul, I would have hi-fived her husband's brutal decision rather than hug and comfort her through many afternoons of sobbing through the pain of her disgrace.

Julian had never been attracted to bright haired blondes with the pseudo-perfect display Karen paraded. Nevertheless, her ridiculously lean, yet cunningly curvy physique was a far cry from the 200 plus pounds I carried on my 5 foot 4 inch frame while moping around with marital stress in the house that would soon become hers. She and Julian had obviously felt an attraction which no one else had seemed to recognize, including myself. And as our marriage grew worse, Karen grew better at building their heartfelt moments while awaiting the perfect moment to grasp what he and I had let go of for far too long.

On the other hand, after three years of being divorced, I'd become excellent at convincing myself I wasn't bitter about their beautifully buff life together which continued to grow in bliss inside my former home. Although it was a great house, I was the one who decided it could no longer be a home to Emily and me after the permanent visual scar of catching them disgustingly making out in the kitchen Julian and I had custom designed for our once happy life together.

Despite the guilt and shame nagging me over and again in losing my marriage, I was still a bit proud I hadn't completely lost myself. Every enormous pound of me was still me. I wasn't rail thin or fabulously fit when Julian and I met years ago in grad school at the Baylor University gym that became our refuge while attempting to get rid of the undergrad pounds which had left us both so frustrated. Even more, being that he absorbed the perpetual drama of my life surrounding my issues with my weight, before and after marrying me, I wasn't driven to continue on in my many failed attempts to be flawlessly fit. The jerk vowed before the two of us, our families, and even God that he would indeed love and support me for better or for worse. Who was I to know that the better to worse would change from pleasantly plump to hideously huge?

"Whitty! Are you even listening to me?" Barb fussed with a laugh.

"Yes! And, the next time you use that now forbidden version of my name, I will use yours too, Barbie!" I laughed in frustration as she interrupted another episode of my daydreaming down memory lane.

Barbie was a name my first cousin seriously wasn't fond of although Aunt Catherine had endearingly named her according to the theme of her childhood nursery. This was another hilarious example of the eccentric nature of Aunt Catherine which Barb had never been good at understanding. Even so, it was apparent to all who knew Barb that my aunt had an uncanny foreshadowing of the fact that the peculiar name would fit her well as she would in reality continue to emerge year after year as a beautiful and ridiculously perfect Barbie doll replica, even after years of marriage and the birth of 8-pounder twin boys.

Barb was 5 feet and 8 inches of lean and lovely perfection with a beautifully chaotic mess of long and curly light brown hair which pulled nothing away from her electric smile and bright brown eyes. My porcelain white Aunt Catherine said that if she'd known her choice to marry a gorgeous black man would've brought forth such a beautiful creation as their daughter, she and Uncle Steve would've bore Barb much sooner. Oh, and she would've birthed at least eight more replicas of her directly afterward.

None could disagree, as Barb was a stunning blend of color as well as beauty. Even when she entered the gym without a trace of makeup, she was still as annoyingly alluring as she was at a formal event when multiple women, including myself, tried their damnedest not to seem as if they were the ugly stepsisters overshadowed by her Cinderella figure while she owned the room floating about in her gorgeousness and genuine charm. Furthermore, much like Cinderella and Barbie's perfect persona, even when she was pushed to her brink, Barb shined as beautiful and radiant on the insice as she clearly was on the outside.

"You know that 'Whitty' was Julian the Jerk's pet name for me! Then again, it's the only matter where his reasoning was just right. It is a perfect blend of my pretty name and perky personality, isn't it?" I chirped with my usual blend of mockery and resentment towards him and myself. "It's just so unfortunate that such an awesome combo wasn't enough to keep him content or faithful."

"Whit, I know it's still difficult, but you and I both know that rehearsing the worst of the pain won't make it go away. You still have so much to be so grateful for in so many of the good things that's occurred between you guys. That includes Emmy, and it includes the fact we all know what a great dad he is to her, and how he still looks after you. Even through the entire breast cancer scare he was right by your side," she attempted to explain in her grandeur gratitude mode. "Julian isn't a careless guy who just set out to stupidly hurt you. He also had to..."

"I can't believe you can still easily defend him!" I interrupted her furiously. "Barb, he cheated on me! Cheated! In our home! Now, he's building a fabulous new life there with the despicable tramp whom you and I practically grew up with," I hissed as every bit of the hurt and humiliation seemed to resurface all over again. "As for the breast cancer scare, it probably would've never happened if it hadn't been for the stress of the damned divorce he eventually threw us over the ledge towards. Sure, his stupid affair happened after a long process of our no longer communicating and all the other difficult crap that marriages simply go through. But he had the nerve to..."

"To what, Whit, try? Because he tried for years. I don't agree with or defend what he did with Karen. It was awful. It was absolutely awful, but he tried his best to help you and to seriously save your marriage. Nowadays, he's still a strong support to both you and Emily. I think it's still a bit tough for you to see what even your therapist is still trying to communicate to you," she attempted to explain herself with sincerity as she frequently did. "It went both ways, Whit. You shut him out. Completely. And, you shut him out far longer than any of us thought you would. You fought him fiercely, and you fought anyone else who seemed to support his efforts to help you for that matter," she continued.

"Thanks, Barb! Please remind me of how wonderful it was to have my entire family and most every friend of mine join in with my lovingly determined jackass husband to get me out of Fatsoland!" I exclaimed, throwing up my arms in a rhythmic frustration. "Oh, she's a chunker! Oh, hide the cupcakes! Oh, she's eating so much! Oh, help her Dr. Fix the Fatties!"

"Dr. Fix the Fatties? You're such a nut, Whit!" Barb retorted with a few uneasy chuckles. "And, you're once again omitting the fact that Julian and the rest of your family were freaked out because your health was in a complete uproar. It's still not fully okay, Whit. You were having bouts of sleep apnea, and you'd just been diagnosed as prediabetic. Now... you are diabetic, unfortunately," she stammered on. "And, let's not forget all the complications you suffered with carrying Emily. Then, almost immediately after having her, your blood pressure issues started. You... you had us all terrified."

"Oh! Am I terrifying you now, Barbie?" I jeered as I shoved in the last huge bite of my cheesecake, chomping down with my mouth and eyes opened wide in mockery of her reasoning.

"Okay, let's not do this," Barb pleaded as she often did during our countless disagreements about everything and nothing. "Whit, I'm not trying to fight with you, and I'm not trying to make you feel awful. I'm sorry I even brought everything up, but you know my passion concerning health and specifically the health of our family. You know that..."

"Yes, I know I didn't get your good luck in our family's gene pool," I snapped as I brought the conversation up a few more decibels as only I could do. "And, I also know I refuse to spend the rest of my life hopelessly trying to win the war on losing the rolls of my never-going-to-be-chiseled abs and the bumps on my lumpy ass so I can be a lean, mean, skinny bitch Barbie doll queen like my fabulous first cousin and favorite pain in my fat ass!"

"Omigosh! Enough already, Whitney! If I've told you once, I've told you a thousand times, my life and my body aren't perfect. You of all people know that. So, your lean, mean skinny bitch quips won't ever convince me I'm a freak of nature for working

21

my ass off to take care of my health. Even more, no matter how viciously defensive you are, I'm not going to stop reminding you I don't want to be at your graveside far too early because you've decided your pride is far more important than seriously taking control of your health. We just watched my... my... my own mom do that to herself," she stammered, trying to choke back tears.

"Barb, I'm... I'm sorry. I was so wrong for... I just..." I attempted to regroup us both, realizing my childish rant was ill-timed in light of what she was experiencing in losing my aunt and her mom.

We all struggled to get through the first Christmas without Aunt Catherine. It was less than a year since she'd passed away of heart disease that had gone completely undetected. She often snickered at Barb's concerns about her health, deciding her daughter had grown far too fanatical in her continual sharing of health news and fitness suggestions that could be so beneficial to all of us.

Barb's insights were never taken seriously by my aunt, who felt she wasn't extremely overweight at 5' 7" and 200 pounds, with energy outside of work readily used to look after her grandsons when her busy schedule allowed. Though she smoked, it was mostly limited to a few nightcaps a week depending on how much Uncle Steve was 'working at reworking her nerves'. Yet, as much as she adored her only child, Aunt Catherine became so annoyed with Barb's constant pleading for her to get active. Nonetheless, she'd always transformed their heated encounters into a good laugh later. I was always open to hearing another story from the Barbie reel, as she called it.

Unfortunately, the last episode wasn't so hilarious. Barb was proud to have found the perfect gift for Aunt Catherine's 58th birthday – membership at a local yoga studio and a personalized yoga mat. She had hoped to pique her mom's interest in exercise in a trendy option like yoga, but it wasn't a moment of celebration when Aunt Catherine placed the sleek membership card and designer mat back into the bow-wrapped box with a faint thank you and a wry smile which plainly communicated that Barb could place her beautiful gift in a place where the sun would never shine.

Barely a month later was she found dead in the kitchen, abruptly cut down by a heart attack. It was unbearably awful. Barb was not only her only child but also the only voice of reason for her family's health. Although he was retired from the military, Uncle Steve was as interested in being fit again as he was in getting a root canal. Those were his exact words. His 6 foot tall, 280 pound frame was larger than his animosity for being told what he should do to take care of his career exhausted body.

Even more, his interests now lay entirely in finding the nearest, darkest pub in which to drown the sorrow of losing the only life that had kept him alive, even though they had driven each other crazy at times. It was a new madness for us all as Uncle Steve seemed determined to rack up DUIs, his third one having occurred just weeks ago. The episode left Barb and her affluent legal giant husband, Rick, in a position where even pulling favors probably wouldn't get him out of that one. The shock and despair was even harder to bear as Uncle Steve's neighborhood was split in a raging dispute over whether or not to exile the man who had cleared three of their lawns in the incident as his tires squealed louder than the pain everyone felt for his loss.

"I'll be fine, Whit," Barb responded with unmistakable annoyance and exhaustion. "It's just been a brutal week trying to get to the bottom of this ordeal with Dad again. Now just isn't the time to bicker with you about the choices you and I know that you simply need to power up and make, once and for all."

"I know. And I'm sorry, but you did piss me off. You know that we big girls don't cry; we bite," I replied as I attempted to get her to follow my lead in a brief chuckle.

"You're so silly, Whit," she smirked.

"And about your question earlier—yes, I'm still serious about reaching my fitness goal. No, I'm not going to give up. I've got a great dress in mind to flaunt, and I won't have you showing me up yet again at another unofficial adult prom," I finished with a teasing wink.

CHAPTER TWO

Poor Little Whit Whit

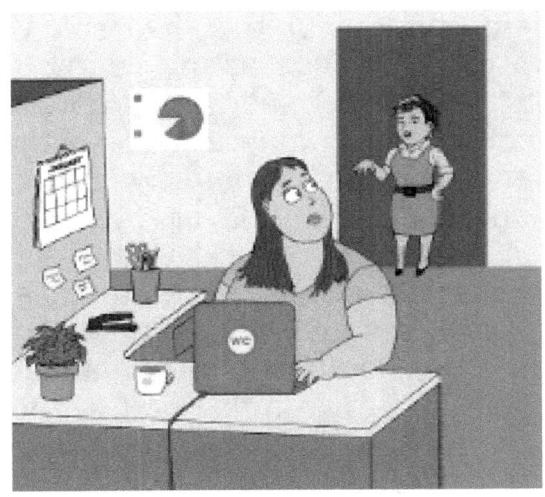

As I scurried about my desk area dreadfully trying to make sure I retrieved what was left of all of my personal belongings, reality with a fine blend of remorse hit yet again. It hit especally hard as I didn't have Barb to talk me through the drive to my unofficial Doomsday since she'd been texting me far more than she'd attempted to return any of my voicemails. She and I clearly knew that when she was too busy to talk, it was because she was too reluctant to tell anyone exactly *why* at that moment. I also knew during our almost delightful lunch the week before, I should've used our time together to have gained her insight on how to deal in my ordeal instead of escalating another silly fight.

My employment at the med spa I'd grown to love with a pride as huge as my yearly bonuses had come to its final end. I spent my final slices of time trying to collect my numerous aching thoughts as I gathered my belongings, fiercely disregarding the constant onset of tears. Over the past weeks, I watched in waves of shock and disappointment, along with the rest of our office staff, as authorities and representatives of various titles and levels of power vigorously completed the mandatory process of rendering Dr. Alcoy's office and services formally worthless in the city of Dallas, or anywhere else in the country for that matter.

I had been the Physician Assistant at La Bella Gente for over five years, however the story was so extensive that even the grittiest of details still weren't completely comprehensive to me. Yet, the bulk of it was clear. There'd been an adequate amount of complaints and confirmations of such to verify that my incredible boss, whom myself and so many others had deemed an amazing doctor, had apparently used his miraculous hands in more ways than necessary on his susceptible patients who one by one mustered the courage to reveal that his sensual methods of remedy had been neither welcomed nor appreciated during his care. Although we the staff knew the well-known secret of Dr. Alcoy having multiple companions outside of the companionship of his marriage, no one had any idea of the extensive nature of his quest for more.

As closely as I worked with him, I could understand why my hideously huge frame had never garnered his inexcusable behavior. Yet, I never gathered that the huge smile beaming through his tall frame and chiseled physique hid such a web of deceit and demise that would cost him his career, his marriage, and his freedom if he were indeed convicted on the charges regarding him.

The years of lavish bonuses and scrumptious holiday and birthday gifts I'd grown to thoroughly enjoy had come to an awful and abrupt end. It ended without any immediate options of severance as the bulk of Dr. Alcoy's assets were in a legal freeze amid multiple negotiations and settlements. Nevertheless, despite the disillusionment and overall dismay, I was grateful I saved a bit for rainy days as I'd learned the valuable lesson of doing so through the drama of my dreadful divorce. I even uncovered a few job leads and secured an actual interview for that upcoming week.

Even so, the idea of starting over and being the new body in the building wasn't anything I felt prepared to pull off all over again. Though my work and reputation had always spoken for itself, another rapid life change felt as if the task would require a lot more energy than I'd be willing or able to provide. Even more, it was tough to grasp the fact I wasn't only losing a terrific job but also the pride I cherished in finally reaching a place in my career

27

that hadn't only provided well for Emily and I but had also given me quite a sense of accomplishment. I lived with the mindfulness of how the crash of my marriage had left me to watch my ex-husband seemingly skip through the rest of his life as I was left to park my own life's details on the curb of despair.

Being financially secure afforded me to refuse the offer of Julian's 'awful alimony'. I called it that without a wink during our volatile divorce proceedings, refusing to accept penance for the piddly apologies he attempted to give in the midst of the pain he caused. Furthermore, I deemed my nuptials address stolen being that I wanted no part of residing where he had initiated his baffling romance. Even so, I insisted as long as he provided well for Emily, his insistence on securing us a new home or furnishing me a monthly stipend laden with guilt wasn't necessary. I felt far more dignity in deciding to pay my own way while pounding the path of happily never after.

"Whit, how much do you have left to go?" Olivia bounced in to ask.

As our office manager, Olivia and I worked just across the foyer from one another for what would have been three years in a month or so. Having had so many good times in the once bustling building, watching her enter my office made it so tough to think back to when it all changed so completely. There was no forgetting the awful moment when she stumbled into my workspace as her signature smile was replaced by a grimaced expression of full-blown tears to alarm me of the buzz that was soon to become national news to all, altering the direction of our lives. Her short salt and pepper hair was a bit disheveled from obviously grabbing at it as she often did in frustration or fun. Even more, the redness in her full cheeks and flat nose told me that her sudden visit to my office to chit-chat was the real deal in *I need to talk to you*.

Olivia had received a call from a friend of a patient who stepped forward after four others had already courageously done so. As many questions as we all initially had concerning the allegations, it was disappointing to realize that quite a few looming inquiries were answered simply in the wake of the news. Having been cheated on myself by a man who I'd thought was a decent husband, I immediately understood why we hadn't seen Dr. Alcoy's wife or two teenaged girls for quite some time. They were active and well-loved fixtures in his establishment, yet they'd been missing like the spa's extra samples of eye creams which no one seemed to know the whereabouts of unless we threatened purse checks or pokes in the eye. We would soon discover that one of the accusers, a friend of the family, had literally taken her allegations to Mrs. Alcoy before formally contacting authorities, and as they say, *it all went downhill from there*.

"I actually have just a few more drawers to empty," I replied, looking up to realize Olivia already had her workout face fully on with the fierceness of her pixie cut roaring at me with more tenacity than the words I knew were coming. The huge spirit which embodied her 4'10" frame was the ultimate example of the quip stating that dynamite comes in small packages.

Olivia had been consistently losing weight and getting her health back in order ever since her son had begun college over a year ago. She decided she no longer wanted to be her version of an unhealthy and unhappy mom, struggling through the day without energy as she tossed through the night without adequate rest. Even more, she longed to be fully active during the empty nest mode of her life, having full energy to adore her new grandson from her daughter and son-in-law. After dropping 35 pounds in the first two months of seriously getting into action, she decided like never before to move forward and never look back. Despite every tough plan of action her trainer required of her and every snack and comfort food I tempted her with, she pushed on with a focus that caused me to further believe that inconsistency is simply a Whitney disease of my exhausted body and brain.

"Whit, you'd better not be moving at a snail pace just to get out of our workout today," she fussed. "I've just gotten back on track over the past couple of weeks because of the crazy holiday season, and I've been sidetracked in taking care of the entire mess here. I can't go back to screwing up my momentum again. You've already bailed on me twice in a row. No more hit and miss. Today is the day, missy. No more excuses. No more..."

"Okay, Deputy Do-right!" I laughed, interrupting her passionate ranting. "I've already told you like eight times that I'm going with you. Besides, I can't blow you off this time being that my official workout buddy is unofficially avoiding me right now. Just give me fifteen more minutes or so to clear these last few drawers and we'll head out."

"What did you do to her this time?" Olivia asked with a raised brow and a slight smirk.

"Wow. So, you automatically think it's my fault? What a friend!" I snickered.

"Whit, I know you. And I've grown to know your roller-coaster relationship with your cousin," Olivia teased. "Really though, what happened? You seem like its weighing heavy on you."

"Argh, I don't know. It was mostly my fault, and I even apologized right after. Barb is just so irritating at times. I mean…"

"The same old clashes?" She interrupted.

"Yes, and I sort of started the thick of it. I snapped on her when she somehow ended up reminding me of why Julian and I didn't work out in regards to *my* decisions about *my* health," I revealed as I stammered through my conflicting thoughts on Barb and I's everlasting ordeal. "She was actually trying to get me onboard the gratitude train as usual, but she just doesn't get it. And, she doesn't completely get me at times."

Being that I only had an older brother, Jason, who'd never been connected to anyone outside of himself and every new girlfriend he picked up, Barb was not only my first cousin but she was also my best friend and only opportunity to have an actual sister from the day she was born. Though I had so

31

much love and admiration for her, I equally harbored just as much frustration. We were rarely on the same wavelength with how we thought or functioned in life, especially in the area of health and fitness. Our relationship underwent many tough walks in the park because of it.

Although Barb was five years my junior, I knew since childhood that I'd never quite measure up to how huge of a deal her tiny frame and huge spirit was amongst our entire family and most of our friends. As the long awaited only child of my Aunt Catherine and Uncle Steve, she was filled with love from her first breath and loved even more for every breath of beauty and positivity she shared with those who absolutely adored her. Though we always kissed and made up after our countless spats surrounding so many issues that were mostly mine, I ended up sinking into more self-hate and sorrow for myself. It was obvious that most of our blowups were a new bout of the old news on the issues of me, me, and me.

Even so, I couldn't imagine Barb would ever get how infuriating it was to try to somehow exist in her glow. It wasn't that I was overcome with full jealously about her lot in life; it was more of a bewilderment of how the hell it had been so ridiculously strenuous most of my life to lose a mere ten pounds, yet I couldn't remember her ever being two pounds overweight. Albeit, I saw the process she endured in the gym, as an adult who bore two kids, to keep her ass firm enough to bounce a full roll of quarters off. I'd always been a reluctant witness of the willpower she maintained while remaining ridiculously consistent in her food choices whether she ate in or out. Even her genuine insight and excitement in the whole process made me reluctantly proud to be officially related to and best of friends with such a fantastic freak of human nature.

It was hard to deal with the fact that her focus and flawlessness had never quite rubbed off on me as I clearly still hadn't figured out how to deal with the ordeal of my weight, despite the many health reports surrounding it and my never-ending frustration about it. It also didn't help that positive cliché upon positive cliché having come from many conversations with Barb constantly swarmed my brain, reminding me that if I somehow gave consistent effort again, I could possibly get the results I craved. Yet, I didn't operate like my annoyingly amazing cousin. She was one of the only people I knew in real life, other than my jackass ex-husband, Julian, who had the stamina and focus to eat damn near perfect and workout religiously, and actually like it.

Though time and again I'd gotten excited and motivated right alongside Barb, the actual agony of the process pushed me out of my progress all over again. Each time I hated myself for quitting again, all the while determining the entire ordeal sucked so bad that quitting felt better than holding on to any sincere hope of one day being able to feel good in my own skin. When would I ever feel good about how I look or how I feel about how I look outside of anyone else's opinion of me?

"Oh, yeah. Barb doesn't get how tough it is for you," Olivia teasingly interrupted my trailing thoughts with her mockery voice used solely for when she felt I was having a pity party. "She doesn't get how long and how hard you've fought. She doesn't get how bad life has been to you in the process. Poor little Whit Whit!"

"Wow! I can't believe I'm going to actually miss your abuse," I laughed in slight embarrassment. "I know you don't like me having any pity parties whatsoever Olivia, but can you at least pretend to be nice to me? Especially on a day like this one."

"Oh, nice. Like you pretend to be to Barb," she continued to tease with seriousness in her voice.

"I am nice to her. It's just difficult to do so when she sits on her throne of fabulously fit perfection reaching down to offer her wonderful advice to me," I shot back. "And, it's not just her, Olivia. This whole mixed up world is set up mostly for the beautiful people with beautiful bodies to live an absolutely beautiful life. I've built a great career based upon this," I continued on, allowing my dam of despair to break. "Yet the fatter my ass becomes, the further away I remove myself from enjoying great clothes which are exclusively made for narrow bodies. Not to mention, the perks in most every influential career that's mostly reserved for picture-perfect frames. Happiness seems to only be enjoyed when you're sparkling happy inside of a hot

34

physique. Barb doesn't get the fact that I've tried my damnedest to follow her useful tips and mimic her steady habits, but the process hasn't worked for me as easily as it's worked for her, ever. I'm so tired of trying to work my huge ass and rolls of flabby abs completely off when all of her parts have been perfectly perfect as long as we can both remember," I grumbled on, staring again at a picture I was packing up from my scrap drawer. "Just look at this picture of us from last summer. Barb is the pinnacle of perfection in her paisley yellow wrap dress, and I... I seriously look like... like I stole someone's favorite blanket and stuffed a few king sized pillows underneath it in that bland khaki dress. It was the only item in my closet that covered the disgust of me without entirely suffocating me last summer," I moaned as I shoved the frame towards Olivia while biting back tears I didn't quite expect to surface. "Look at this crap, and tell me why I should be so happy for all the perfect people prancing around in their perfect bodies!"

"Whit, there's no such thing as a perfect body, no matter which doctor with a delightful team designs it," she winked a smile at me, holding up the picture to view it as best she could without her glasses. "This isn't an awful picture of you, especially with that gorgeous face of yours. Woman, if a perfect body is all you're pushing for in getting the unhealthy weight off, you'll always be in an awful state of unhappiness, even if you put a polished smile on it," she continued smiling with a tone of pure empathy, tempting me to allow my every

35

suppressed tear to fall. "Do you remember that quote about Mother Teresa I shared with you a couple of weeks ago?"

"Oh no, not that craziness again," I laughed. "It's hilarious, but it's hilarious because it's so damn crazy."

"It's so damn true, and I'll repeat it again," Olivia giggled before repeating the quote she'd found on Pinterest. "Mother Teresa didn't go about life complaining about her thighs. She had stuff to do. Whit, your losing weight has got to be about much more than trying to measure up to a perfection that never has and never will exist. You have an amazing career to grow. You have a beautiful daughter to raise. You have people all around you who need you to be healthy and whole, and full of energy because your life matters in their lives. Life is barren when we allow the anticipated applause of our physique to exceed the strength of our spirit. Wake up, my friend."

"I am awake. I'm just wide awake now to realize how hard this process has been for me as long as I can remember," I retorted with even more despair.

"Need I remind you that the process hasn't worked easily for me? Hola, mi amiga divertida! My 49-year-old body has had to work the hell out of this once rusty frame!" She laughed, throwing in her Spanglish words to amusingly keep my attention. "It's been a challenge for me from day one, chica, and I'm sure it's been a challenge for Barb. Getting fit is tough for everyone, just on different levels. It only gets better as you decide over and again to use all of that frustrated energy to keep yourself moving instead of hating on whoever you think may have it so much easier or better than you do."

"Hating on! When did you become so cool?" I laughed out loud.

"It's called learning to stay connected to your college kid far beyond your credit card support. Just wait until Emily grows up. You'll learn more than you ever thought you needed to know," she laughed. "And don't miss the point I'm trying to make to you. You can't keep on giving up on yourself, Whit. You're so good at convincing yourself that the people who're actually pulling for you are somehow pouncing on you when they're actually trying to help in the best ways they know how. Don't forget, I was over 200 pounds last year, and I haven't lost 55 pounds and counting by focusing on the crazy stuff. Now, I'll be back in a few more minutes after I load my car and then we're out of here, okay?" She smiled.

I nodded in reluctant agreement as I smiled back at Olivia and realized once again how much I'd grown to really appreciate the friendship and camaraderie she and I seemed to build from day one, despite our huge difference in age and upbringing. At 49 years of age she was twelve years my senior, yet the connection between us mostly felt like a long-lasting high school friendship rather than an elder taking a minor under her wing. Her hilarious Spanglish and fiery Latino warmth reminded me of my dad's entire family, thus I knew the heavens had smiled on me personally when Olivia took the office management opening at La Bella Gente after her husband's job moved their family from Mesa, Arizona to the official south in Dallas. Paul's lucrative oil executive income didn't require her needing to work at all, yet God himself clearly knew I would desperately need her relentless wisdom and wit during the reconstruction of some of the most challenging times I'd ever imagined seeing in my life.

Nonetheless, as much as I loved and appreciated Olivia and her wisdom, she was no Aunt Catherine. I had no doubt in my soul that if only my amazing aunt were still around to be my exclusive mentor and advisor, the mental battle I suffered in the mess of a messy job transition would've been seized immediately. I actually pursued my career field in Dermatology having seen Aunt Catherine's happiness and success in the plastic surgery field. Long before it was completely accepted or popular to pinch and poke until we got it just right with our physical attributes and appearances, she was doing a wonderful job and making a wonderful life at it.

Though I still had my own mommy dearest, my relationship was still as it had always been with Mom. I loved her. I hated her. I was always trying to love her again, hoping she'd stop saying and doing the outrageously annoying and hurtful things which made me hate her just a bit more. That was during a pretty good week with us, as I was apparently too much of a living reminder of who Dad was and who he wasn't in our lives.

It had been almost eight years since we lost Dad due to complications with Type II diabetes. The fact that he was only 51 years old when he died of kidney failure brought on by the progression of his diabetes had never settled well with my super fit mom who was always on his case to take care of his health. Dad spent years of eating everything he felt he deserved to eat while refusing to do anything he didn't feel like doing. Mom overly reprimanded and reminded him that his choices would ultimately shorten his years and cause us all more pain and grief than his excessive weight caused him to endure.

His death was too much for our family to accept individually or together. I was not only a complete daddy's girl, but I was also the heir apparent of his bad genes. Every issue that obesity brought to his body began to surface in mine even before Dad died, as my weight continuously increased. Mom made it clear through her actions and non-action towards my brother and I that it was beyond infuriating to have her daughter with a foot pointed toward the grave while her son, whose grief and anger over Dad being in the grave, hadn't brought his feet back to our family home since the funeral. Jason blatantly believec Dad's untimely death was partly due to the condescending bickering of Mom. Thus, we all avoided the depth of those conversations, accepting the fact we hadn't much love left for one another or the family we no longer had.

Albeit, Mom swore she loved me despite our back and forth bashing sessions spewing with her unsolicited advice about my health and life's details, all underlined with her internal judgment deeming I'd never be enough until I'd lost enough weight. Consequently, it was beyond tough to believe any statement of her of love as it seemed to crush her heart that I retained all of her beautiful features except her 5' 6", 130 pound frame that paraded a nonexistent waist and firm ass which I hadn't even possessed in my high school years.

Though I often received compliments on my beauty with my long locks of full brown hair framing a fairly olive and virtually flawless face, nothing about my beauty felt beautiful. Despite the fact that my glistening green eyes and full lips were displayed on a face void of an *I'll be entering my 40's soon* message, I felt as attractive as Humpty Dumpty shoved into a spandex dress. Though I spent years wisely following methods of excellent care for my skin, I idiotically failed time and again to take care of my 5 foot 4 inch frame which was obviously tugging over 250 pounds. The despair in enduring a body whose negligence can't be ignored past a pretty face is more difficult to describe than explaining another bad day at work. I hated it, and I hated myself for allowing my body to get to the point of hating it.

Furthermore, knowing my 60-year-old mom's fabulously fit frame was as impressive as my Barbie doll cousin confirmed the unfairness and misery of my lot in life. Not to mention, Barb actually enjoyed my mom in a way I would never understand just as I had enjoyed hers. Although she and I were roughly five years apart and of completely different racial backgrounds, with my mom marrying a Latino man, while her mom, my aunt, married a Black man, Barb hilariously insisted we were somehow cosmically switched at birth. However, since we were clearly sisters anyway, it shouldn't matter to investigate it much. Being that I'm the elder of us, she'd rather I bring my gray hairs in by fretting about something more important than the revelation of such a plot. All of that craziness was Barb's exact words.

All in all, no matter how my weight unpredictably inflated or deflated, Aunt Catherine had loved and empathized with me through every crazy stage, often asking few questions or explanations about any of it. She simply cheered me on at my heaviest and happy danced with me in every short-lived victory of leaning out just enough to squeeze into another event driven outfit. Each time I needed a quick stitch or unstitch in my couture to accommodate the fluctuations in my weight, she was always willing to take on the role as my secret seamstress. Through every crash and burn of every yo-yo diet or fad I found and loved with pride and then dropped with humiliation, she was always proud of the real me in the midst of all the madness and fluctuating pounds.

"Ok, ready or not, vamos! We can get changed at the gym," Olivia announced, taking her stance in my doorway again. "And, I've already grabbed a stash of everything I think we'll both need and enjoy from the foyer cabinets."

"Aren't you just so helpful?" I laughed, knowing she had taken on that task to prevent any further delay of mine in getting us on to the gym.

"I sure am," she teased back. "And, just so you know, I'm only carrying the smallest of your items to your car. You can carry the rest of it as part of your warm up for our session today."

"You're such a thoughtful friend, Olivia!" I laughed in a sugary sarcastic tone.

"Tu sabes!" She teased again in Spanish.

"Yes, I do know it. And, I appreciate it, mi amiga," I responded in laughter. "Let's go get our punishment!"

CHAPTER THREE

A Way with Words

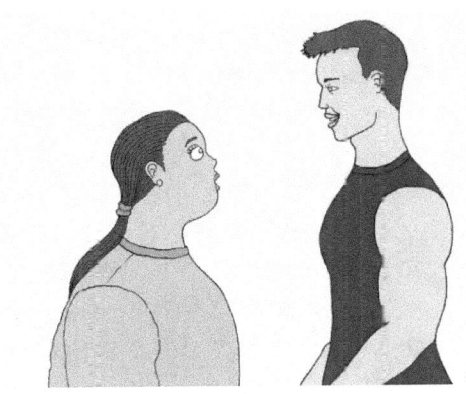

Although I always made sure to bring in a current gossip magazine issue to help me get through my all too frequent fight on the elliptical, I was still panting ridiculously in frustration and hoping that the 18 minutes displayed on that shiny console was my time done, rather than the time remaining. The first intervals of my workouts were always the hardest as I contemplated whether or not to simply call it quits while my shortness of breath and my irritable brain tried to figure out why the hell I was deciding to take my body onto another trip of torture. The ultimate misery of the misery was that I wasn't finding any motivation to convince myself of the payoff of another sweaty session despite the goals I'd already declared to Barb and myself. The more I pondered upon the details of my life, the more I realized I simply didn't have any real enthusiasm to do the work I knew it would take to once again get to a point where my agony in working out would actually become an enjoyable part of my day again and ultimately get me to the results I so desperately needed.

I had barely lost six pounds since I finally tucked away my holiday season habits, and I had at least 20 more pounds to go in order to get to a point where I could actually stand myself in even a few of the outfits I had in mind for Barb's spring event only a few short months away. The mere thought of knowing if I totally bailed on my goals that I'd be forced to show up to another spring event looking like the huge bunny hiding an extra bundle of Easter eggs made me more frustrated than standing in a long line awaiting my caramel whipped lattes.

I'd already begun to do my combination of hoping and moping as my split personality of reasoning kicked into high gear yet again. If I could lose at least 20 pounds, maybe I wouldn't completely hate myself as I bailed on my real hope of actually losing 40 pounds overall—the hope of 40 pounds in less than 12 weeks. Although I was trying to process the hilarity of my somehow kicking in the discipline to ever see it happening, it was my actual goal. Notwithstanding, the awfully honest part of me knew I'd have to seriously struggle and scrape to lose every bit of the 20 pounds I'd pressure myself to lose, and then celebrate like it was my actual aspiration, only to quickly gain every pound back as I basked in a 'reward myself' excitement of losing anything to begin with.

Even worse was the fact I truly couldn't imagine spending another spring season in utter frustration as a 250 pound plus fat ass while beginning the dreadful process of taking off the layers of clothes a brief winter season fortunately allowed to cover up the truth of every ripple and roll of me. I sickened with anxiety about the coming arrival of another hot summer of wearing long and flowing frocks which felt like blankets in the blistering summer heat of Dallas. It was my futile attempt to hide a body that in so many ways I could no longer bear to reveal in my own privacy.

"Hey, how's your heart rate, Whit?" Olivia interrupted my exhausting thoughts, calling over to me in full smiles while apparently enjoying her agony on the stair climber. She'd been learning about heart rate training over the past couple of months, thus she was constantly attempting to practice her new-found expertise on me each time she had an opportunity to do so. With the known issues I had with high blood pressure, she had the inkling her insight was so incredibly useful.

"I'm actually going to go and refill my water bottle before EMS ends up being my official escort out of here this afternoon," I laughed in irritation, stepping a bit too hastily off the left side of the elliptical and landing completely on my huge ass—the ass already worn out from the few minutes of painful effort that slaughtered me.

My attempt to prevent my awful thud or anyone from seeing it was pointless. Before I knew it, the floor was my home as I fought to change my address immediately. I sat scrambling uncontrollably to get up when Olivia leaped off the stair master squealing in complete hilarity and shock, shuffling to my aid. I cackled in disbelief and disgrace, frantically grasping to get up before gym management would be forced to call in a crane for support, or an inconspicuous cell phone user would have an opportunity of a lifetime to present the best viral video ever captured in a North Dallas gym.

"Wow! I guess you really are trying to get EMS in here today, aren't you?" She teased as I reached out to her hands in frustrated determination, longing to run to the nearest private break spot or a buried cave as soon as my ass left that gym turf.

Even in our riotous laughter, I wanted to not only disappear permanently into the spot I was obviously stuck in on the floor but also run full force out of the main doors never return to it again. Of course my lists of degrees and certifications didn't prepare me for acts of illusion, and a full force run wasn't coming out of my thunder thighs plastered to the ground. Nonetheless, my few minutes on that evil elliptical was far more devastating than my mortifying crash.

"I'm okay!" I responded to the worried expression covering Olivia's face beyond our giggles, as it took quite a bit of effort to help me up.

"Are you sure? I'm totally okay with cutting my workout a bit short and getting us out of here. Of course that won't be before we demand a complete apology from this elliptical for deliberately attacking you for no apparent reason," she chuckled, attempting to make me laugh a bit more in light of the humiliation plastered on my face.

"I don't know how you missed your calling as a stand-up comedian, silly woman," I snickered, brushing off my workout pants as I stood up and looked past her shoulders for the nearest water fountain. "I'll be okay. Just finish up your fun on your ridiculous machine. I need to get completely away from mine for a few moments to find some well needed hydration," I muttered, walking away briskly yet feebly from the scene I'd made.

To acd insult to every bit of injury my body and soul felt, a few seconds into my quest for rest and recovery from my shameful blunder, I was enthusiastically interrupted by a buff and beaming trainer who seemed to be drinking in the positivity punch at Dynamo Fitness.

"How's it going today?" He grinned. His smile looked a bit familiar, yet I didn't know him being that my presence at the gym was often as solid as a nail in a hollow wall.

Despite my initial thoughts of excitement upon joining months before, even the remarkable aesthetics and positive atmosphere at Dynamo hadn't conquered my battle to stay on the consistency train. With its brightly painted walls and trendy music bellowing just enough to entertain everyone who walked into the lobby, it was hard not to even slightly smile when greeted by the happy faces at the front desk seeming to enjoy the arrival of every guest. With every piece of exclusive workout equipment one could imagine on a workout floor along with a wide-ranging list of group fitness classes in impeccable rooms welcoming even the most hesitant eye to peek in on the action, I couldn't quite understand why I'd much rather spend my designated workout time on one of the soft leather couches in the pristine locker room or even huddled away with a good book in one of the cozy armchairs in the full service café. It would've been even better to escape to the outside pool which was more magnificent than anything inside the massive building, however I couldn't imagine marching my massive frame out there to relax in the resort atmosphere. There was no way I was taking my beach whale of a body for a swim amongst some of the best bodies I'd seen on many of the faces I cared for in Dallas. It was tough enough seeing the fit and fabulous everywhere else throughout the fancy framework of Dynamo.

"How do you think it's going?" I thought with annoyance, returning his enthusiastic greeting with a half-snarled smile. There I was limping to the water fountain and contemplating a bolt directly to the

48

main doors, yet he was grinning as if we were both in our happy places. The only thing stopping me from actually making a run for it was the long walk I knew I'd have to hike back to my car as I'd made myself carpool with Olivia to ensure I completed my visit.

"It's just great. Can't you see the specks of glitter glowing through my sweat beads today?" I retorted as I felt his eagerness to greet anyone in such obvious agony as mine deserved a saucy sarcasm.

"Hmm. Yeah. I thought I saw a fairy dust of some sorts trailing not too far behind you," he laughed in response.

"Wow, you may be just as brave as you are nuts," I shot back with a snarly smirk. "I take it you don't really know the intensity of a woman who's fuming as I am from a tough and unfinished battle with the elliptical."

"Oh, I've seen some things inside these walls. You must've been doing the hill training program. That one definitely gets your heart rate going," he smiled, reaching out his hand to fully introduce himself. "I'm Cory, and you are?"

"I'm Whitney," I replied with an actual excitement to shake his hand despite the disturbance that led me towards his direction. "And no, I wasn't doing the hill training mode. I was actually doing the kill myself to rebuild myself mode. I think that one is Level 14 in my manual, and I'm sure Level 2 in yours," I continued with even more snarkiness in efforts to hide the embarrassment quickly kicking in from my being so exhausted with the entry level manual mode I hadn't even completed.

He laughed, continuing his chatter with a genuine concern I wouldn't have expected to match a personal trainer of his appearance. His 6 foot 3 inch frame was assembled with muscles exuding through every fiber of the fitted compression tee he wore so well. The dazzling smile radiating from his full lips had me totally nervous to utter another word to him yet completely comfortable to want to continue on chatting with him the rest of my entire Saturday afternoon. However, as I sized up his chiseled frame and took in his warm smile as bright as his full hair was dark, I made a quick note to self to get my fluttered heart together. I knew he could see past my flawless face right to my bulging body and decide what quite a few hotties decided about me: what a beautiful face, but as for a great body, no. And, no thank you.

I frequently saw the reaction during gatherings and interactions of all kinds, coming even from guys whom I wouldn't have considered having a connection with if they were the last guy in the shallow pool of available men. Nonetheless, I knew how to face the fact that the only hot factor concerning me was the brush fire my thighs often threatened as they rubbed together profusely while fighting to move forward in my every step. Though I'd connected with a couple of good guys since my dreadful divorce, those who seemed to be interested

50

beyond my body or lack thereof quickly retreated in disinterest as my obvious issues with my large physique came to surface faster than bees swarm to a honeycomb.

It was becoming harder to deal as my 5'4" frame was now over 250 pounds. My heart was more distraught about it than my brain was exhausted in figuring out how to decide what to do about it, considering the back and forth steps taken with my weight as long as I could remember. With my blood pressure and sleep apnea issues, I didn't want to risk undergoing weight loss surgery, even if it would bring an overnight transformation to my body accustomed to many long nights of overeating. Even more, the scare I'd overcome months ago in discovering that the huge tumor in my huge breasts wasn't actually cancerous was enough reason for me to stay away from all medical procedures outside of my skin treatments. Besides, the already long lists of checkups scheduled for doctors and specialists all over North Dallas was more than I could handle in my life reconstruction project.

"Are you at least getting the results you want Whitney, or does everything seem to be remaining the same?" Cory interrupted my frustrating thoughts.

"It depends on what you mean by results. Albeit, I'm sure your definition of results is connected to your shrewd personal trainer lingo to persuade me to ask about what you provide in physical punishment only meant to drain my bank account as I ultimately annoy your nerves, refusing to completely give in to your helpful tips and torment," I challenged him with a flirtatious defiance which surprised me despite the nervousness I felt.

"Wow, you certainly have a way with words," Cory laughed out loud again.

"Oh, there's more from where that came," I shot back in my sugary sweet and sarcastic tone. "Especially since it's obvious by the overall zest in your greeting and expressions that you seem to actually believe what's going on in here is somehow enjoyable."

"Oh, it can become gratifying when the time spent here is effective, and you're getting adequate results," he responded with a tone in his voice as tranquil as he was attractive and a slightly serious expression to convey his talking to me rather than at me.

"Oh, results again. Well, I've lost about 10 pounds in the last month or so," I lied as I dared not confess my six pounds lost since the wrap up of the holiday season. Even more, the accomplishment was more from a quick reform rather than consistent effort. I had cut back on eating out twice a day knowing my lifestyle would be changing a bit financially in leaving La Bella Gente. "So, I guess I am making progress."

"That's definitely progress," he affirmed. "Do you have a bigger goal in mind?"

"Oh, is it that obvious?" I laughed as I looked up and down at myself cleverly teasing my heavy frame, as I'd grown so good at doing in attempt to defuse the annoyingly shameful frustration of it.

"Good one, but that's not what I meant," he chuckled. "I've just found the vast majority of people in here aren't looking to lose just a few pounds or so. There's often a bigger goal in minc. Whether it's an actual event, a wakeup call due to an event, or some other reason keeping you motivated pass the—what did you call it, torment?"

"Yes, torment," I laughed in slight embarrassment yet admiration, realizing he'd been indeed listening to my every word. "The only reason I'm allowing you to continue talking my head off is because I don't quite feel like returning to the remainder of my torment on an elliptical that literally attacked me. But yes, I actually do have a bigger goal in mind, not that I'll actually accomplish it."

"Hmm. If you don't mind my asking, what do you mean by 'Not that I'll actually accomplish it'? Is it a crazy outrageous goal or are you actually not allowing yourself full confidence to get after it?" He inquired further with full eye contact, causing me to smile and swoon simultaneously.

"Well, a bit of both I guess. The specific amount I have in mind isn't outrageous, but it's more than I've challenged myself to do at once in quite some time. So, I'm just keeping my excitement level subtle enough so if I don't completely reach my ultimate goal, I won't tear myself up about it in the aftermath," I shared with him without thought he'd decipher anything further from my well-rehearsed response I'd successfully convinced my own brain of.

"Oh, so let me make sure I understand you. Your goal is actually doable. It's even what you really want. However, you're going to spend a little bit more effort in preparing yourself not to hit your mark so when you do fail, as you'll be prepared to do so, your heart will take it a bit easier by not having become so excited in the first place about what you truly wanted to accomplish to begin with," he peered at me through his glistening green eyes with a smile informing he saw completely to the heart of my insanely defeating reasoning.

"I guess you don't miss anything, do you, Cory? How did I even get to the point of discussing all of this with you?" I responded with a *please don't completely humiliate me* smile.

"I just tend to call it as I see it when someone gives me the ear to do so, Whitney. Furthermore, you're discussing it because you sense this chit-chat is a safe zone, as it really is," he smiled with the assurance he wasn't trying to humiliate me.

"So, being that you're the actual expert, what wildly brilliant tips can you quickly give me to start reaching my goals?" I teased to deflect from my defeated gibberish.

"I actually don't tend to work with random tips or on-the-go haste, Whitney," he laughed. "I've found the individuals who're really serious about not only reaching their fitness goals but also making a real life change want stable results. That generally takes more than a quick chit-chat or a three to five step instant miracle plan."

"Oh, so you're saying I'd probably have to spend most of my life and loads of my money with you in order to one way or another become a healthy, happy, perfect me," I tested him with my trusty sarcastic shield fully on.

"I'm not saying that at all," he smirked at my sarcasm as he continued on. "From only a brief conversation, I wouldn't immediately suggest what type of training would be the best component for you initially or long-term. Before we'd discuss anything farther than your next two steps, I'd have to discover by way of an actual assessment where your physical starting point is in relation to where you say you ultimately want to go. However, I'm not so sure you're completely certain of what direction you actually wart to go right now, except maybe out of this now seriously serious conversation, I'm sure," he teased a bit as we both smiled at the nature of our conversation even more.

"I'm okay with a serious chit-chat. I'm a Physician's Assistant in Dermatology. Much of my daily conversation consists of serious moments of giving answers to even seriously silly questions at times," I laughed, barely mustering up a decent reply amidst his observations that seemed to have so much insight into areas I was so good at masking. "But, an assessment? Ha-ha! That would probably blow both our minds!"

"Really, how so?" He searched intently with another a solid smile.

"Cory, I've had enough doctor visits and completed questionnaires to fill two lifetimes. They all advise me of the same thing. Get healthy. Get it together. Do it now. As if it isn't what I've been trying to do this entire time," I finished with my familiar exhaustion.

"Hmm. So, where do you believe the disconnection is occurring?" He asked with a concern I couldn't ignore.

"Hmm. It's probably between my fridge, my pantry and my constant frustration with the lack of results I have to live with over and again. All because I have far more enjoyment in putting calories into my body than going through the strenuous and sweaty routine of getting them out," I laughed. "If I could just wake up one day and no longer have to go through this awful process of struggling to keep my favorite foods from adding to my ever growing waistline, I'm sure life would be as wonderful for me as a skinny bitch at Fashion Week. But, that's not the case, so I'll just take my lot in life and work with what I've got, no matter how heavy it continues to get."

"Oh, I see. So does your 'lot in life' have an open ear for maybe a suggestion or two?" He chuckled with no attempt to conceal his concerned expression.

"Go ahead. I'm a big girl. We big girls don't cry; we bite," I grinned as he laughed out loud at my trademark joke which had always gotten under my ex-husband's skin.

"Have you ever thought about utilizing the energy you have to express a little more hope for yourself instead of simply dwelling on your frustrations? It's definitely true that everyone's lot in life isn't to be a naturally, how did you say it, 'skinny bitch'? But, with all due respect, Whitney, most all of the info you've given me on yourself hasn't been much to suggest you have a great deal of hope in getting what you say you want. In a cynical mindset like the one you've expressed, I've seen that even the most phenomenal fitness plans won't yield any lasting change or results for that individual," he spoke with a confidence and compassion that was in my face yet seemingly at my side to support me. "You can take or leave my feedback if you like. I've just found it's helped so many to consider that a huge part of what we're able to accomplish physically begins or ends with the positive mental strength we choose to cultivate or neglect."

"Wow. So, I guess my workout is completely over after that swift kick in the throat," I laughed in embarrassment, yet with an odd sense of gratitude.

"Whitney, your workout was over when you came limping over to that water fountain in frustration," he teased. "Really though, I hope you've heard the essence of what I've said and not just the wordage."

"Oh, I've heard the essence of it. That's why I'm thinking that I may have to change gyms now,

Cory. I can't show my pretty face in a place where someone felt it necessary to rip me bare and reveal some of the nitty-gritty truths to my saga," I teased him with a comfort I hadn't felt with a genuinely hot guy in quite some time. "I know it's Saturday, but is your manager around so I can also thank him personally for your wonderful words and insight?"

"I'm actually his Assistant Manager, but he wouldn't be surprised about your gratitude at all. I may still be on his top ten list of fix-it's with customer feedback," he teased back at me with another huge laugh. "But on a more serious note, when you fully decide to map out a solid plan for your goals, I'd certainly be interested in taking care of an assessment for you to help you begin to design a program that will work specifically for you. Let me give you one of my cards," he continued while reaching in his back pocket to hand me his business card. "My schedule can get a bit hectic at times, but I'm flexible."

"Okay. I'll consider it," I smirked as I accepted the card. "As soon as I convince myself to take on a little more punishment, I'll head your way."

"I look forward to seeing you around," he smiled with an odd look of optimism as I began to head back to rejoin Olivia for what I hoped was the wrap up of our cardio time.

CHAPTER FOUR

Fight or Fit

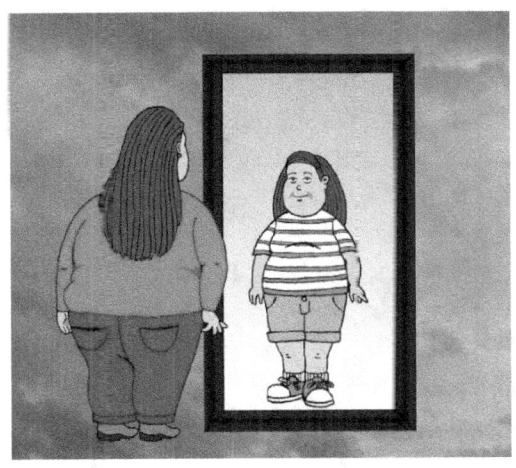

"**M**orning Whitney! Are we having a good day so far?" Kristina beamed in with her trademark smile, increasingly causing me to wonder whether it was truly who she was, or if Dr. Carson had pumped smiley gas into her lip injections that she was slightly more proud of than the '*70 pounds and counting*' she continually announced as having lost over the past six months.

Kristina had been Dr. Carson's PA for four years. She was more than thrilled and supportive when I came on as Dr. Thomas' new PA. His previous, Carol, took a maternity leave which ended up being a full exit of her career, choosing to remain home and raise her twin girls. Though we were complete opposites in many ways, Kristina and I became immediate friends as her congenial personality made it impossible not to accept her welcome mat of camaraderie. I'd heard her ongoing inspirational weight loss story more times during my mere month at Radiant Reveals than I'd cheated on every miracle diet in my entire lifetime. Though I was as happy for her as my own exhausted life in trying to get fit could be, I was happier when she wasn't giving me every detail of her so amazing fitness journey while I continually tried to fully kick-start my own ass into gear, only to kick myself later as I'd quit again as fast as I restarted.

Kristina wasn't the only one who beamed with happiness and positive energy in my new professional world. Even our slightly underpaid aestheticians chirped with encouraging clichés and greetings to each other and every client throughout our brightly decorated spa laden with white cabinetry and modern furniture. The bright space was understandably warm in our optimistic atmosphere. Dr. Carson and Dr. Thomas alike smiled at everyone more than I was accustomed to amongst MD's, and both their wives carried in cheeseball smiles and oodles of happiness, popping in from time to time. My month or so at Radiant Reveals quickly began to feel like too many years of too many smiles, too many happy greetings, and too many positive meetings of way too much wonderful insight on how to live a radiant life inside out.

Though I was thankful to secure a sound position after the crash and burn of La Bella Gente, I wasn't completely happy it landed me in an over-the-top happy land which not only thrived off loads of positive energy but also a seriously strong mindset that a fit and healthy body is a significant key to happiness in our lives. It was an absolute miracle of misery for my heavy body and mostly unhappy mind to withstand. Barb said it could definitely be the best scenario for my life at the moment, therefore I was thinking in ungrateful terms by becoming increasingly annoyed with it all. Then again, my freakishly health driven cousin would certainly fit well into such an alternate universe, especially as their love for all things fit proved as fanatic as hers.

Each week at the spa was reminder after annoying reminder of how dreadful it is to eat unhealthy and attempt to function without consistent exercise. Top that with multiple mentions on how fantastic it is to live fit and frolic about with happy smiles and purses loaded with healthy snacks. It was irritating to see everyone's hands frequently wrapped around fresh fruit smoothies undoubtedly blended with a surge of mind-bending positive energy.

I was aware that my annoyance with the details exaggerated them just a bit. My unofficial big sister and mentor, Olivia, lovingly reminded me so each time I sent a quick text her way about my appalling new job plusses. She suggested I take a chill pill in such a fortunate atmosphere, but I told her I was already taking far too many pills for the issues that circulated through my heavy frame. I couldn't believe such a great career opportunity would give me more nauseating reasons to be annoyed at every reminder of what I just couldn't seem to do about my pounds and pounds of weight, and the woes that accompanied it.

I hadn't been to the gym in almost two weeks as I'd taken yet another unofficial break. It was mostly an attempt to avoid that hunk of a trainer, Cory, after our insightful conversation. Each time I'd seen his 6 foot 3 inches of smiles and way too sexy muscles, it reminded me of what I really wasn't doing in Dynamo Fitness: building a fit frame. It also reminded me of what I'd most likely never have: a healthy life with a hot guy. I just couldn't get my shit together. Even more, I was far too exhausted and too frustrated to care about it at times. While my fairly fabulous face kept me in the dating circle, I was the big girl whose pretty face could land the attention of most any handsome guy, yet whose body stopped the love train abruptly, seeming like a giant sized joke alongside him.

Barb reminded me that my mental views about myself weren't healthy, constantly advising it's as important to get my mental shape in tow while striving to get the excess weight off. Of course this was coming from a darling woman who'd never carried an extra pound in her life and didn't have the slightest idea of what it actually feels like to have real cravings for good food raging on the inside of her. All I really wanted was to get rid of the uncomfortable ton of ripples and rolls on my body, even as I added more pounds to the pressure of it all. Yet, I couldn't get myself to work towards changing any of it, at least not consistently.

"I was hoping we could chat over a couple of things before our hectic afternoon starts," Kristina interrupted my trailing thoughts again with her loads of bright energy and morning chipperness.

"Sure, about what?" I answered, barely making eye contact with her as I forced my face to portray my best smile.

"Well, I want your feedback on an anti-aging facial I'm looking at implementing into our collection in the next couple of weeks. And, I finally picked up a copy of the gluten-free cookbook we chatted about last Tuesday. The one I figured would help me to sustain some solid energy in my next phase of fat loss," she beamed as her long auburn hair covered her smile I could feel radiating throughout my entire office as she searched through her tote bag to reveal her find.

"Oh, the gluten free, *'Bread is bad. Cupcakes are cruel. Eat not, or forever keep your weight.'* cookbook?" I responded with a laugh, attempting to conceal the annoyance building in my throat.

"You're more and more hilarious by the day, Whitney!" Kristina chuckled before sincerely trying to explain her new-found insight as usual. "But no, it's actually not about depriving yourself. It's about eating clean and nutritious food that's still delicious but sure to help us continue to drop the unhealthy and unwanted pounds."

"So, I'm guessing your current weight loss goals aren't only to start shopping with the tweens at Forever 21, but you're also aiming to get your swimsuits at Osh Kosh B' Gosh," I laid on the sarcasm as thick and salty sweet as I could. "Yea! That new cookbook will definitely fit right in with your passion for every power veggie, and your love for super-duper fresh fruit, and maybe even your determination to make sure you drink more water than an Egyptian camel."

"Oh that's not what I meant, Whitney," she responded with a nerved yet nervous look. "Is that what it sounds like, or are you just being sarcastic in a seriously sarcastic manner?"

"It's just a little sweet sarcasm to help me get through another happy day of hearing about how happy life is in Kristina's happy land of happily dropping the weight that took so much happiness from her now truly happy life," I responded with no further attempt to conceal my annoyance.

Though I was mostly glad for Kristina's happiness in living in a completely different body, it was tough to swallow the fact that her continued results placed her moments away from being a physical twin of my Barbie doll cousin, Barb. Although Kristina's long, bone-straight auburn hair framing her round porcelain face and icy blue eyes was completely opposite of Barb's light brown chaotic curls which often buried her narrow caramel toned face and light brown eyes, the story was virtually the same. The 'Your Life Sucks' award was due to be presented to me yet again as another bombshell beauty's consistent progress only reminded me of the over 250 pounds I haphazardly tugged around on my 5'4" frame—the frame I was allowing to increase meal by meal.

"Whoa. My apologies, Whitney. I certainly didn't mean to irritate you with my fitness finds. I thought you liked chatting about the interesting things I'm still discovering in this weight loss process being that you're also pretty determined to get your life back," she replied with complete embarrassment in her voice.

"Interesting. Ok, we're talking interesting," I glared directly at her while continuing in my signature *you asked for it* voice. "Why don't we chat about my interesting run to Domino Donut Shoppe this morning when I had to wait behind two lingering idiots, who happened to be a cute fit couple with no idea of what they had a taste for while I stood there impatiently waiting and wanting to order damn near one of everything in the case knowing my caloric intake for the day has no margin for even a crumb of what was on display," I continued on with pure venom. "Or, we can chat about how interesting it'll be on my upcoming date this weekend as I attempt to explain to another online potential, who I've been excitedly chatting with for weeks, that the pictures he's seen of me is definitely me, but the extra 50 pounds he's seeing in person is my sexy surprise gift to help him show himself an even stronger man if he dares to toss me over his shoulders in complete excitement of meeting me," I grimaced in aggravation and embarrassment of revealing such humiliation to her. "Hopefully, his face will show more humor about it than the disappointment which already resides in my own mind about how I really look."

"Whitney... I had... no idea..." Kristina stammered on as I continued with my bitterly sarcastic diatribe.

"Or even better, let's chit-chat on how interesting it's been to try to figure out how to explain to my 11-year-old Emily that my not wanting to do the upcoming Fun Run with her for her afterschool program isn't because I don't want to have fun with her. It's because I can't even force my fat ass to get motivated to walk around our neighborhood. Attempting to do a 1 and 1/2 mile run would surely be the end of me, and it would be the real beginning of her fully seeing what a huge loser and slacker her mom is compared to her super fit Superman cloned dad and her unofficial stepmom who's apparently training to be another Little Miss Healthy Pants like my irritating cousin who currently holds the supreme crown for that title," I finished with exhausted relief of being real about what I knew everyone really saw about my miserable life in my miserably overweight body.

"Whitney, I had no idea all of this is going on. You've never... never mentioned that..." She fumbled through her response, attempting to continue our exhausting round of chatter. "When... when did you even go back to eating donuts again? I thought you'd erased those completely off of your cheat list."

"After everything I just said, all you can actually focus on is my having donuts this morning?" I laughed at her with full blown annoyance. "Kristina, has your amazing weight loss caused you to totally lose touch with how crazy hard it is to actually eat most of the stuff we call healthy? I've been eating that sawdust tasting oatmeal you're so in love with for breakfast over the past week and a half. I needed a doughnut this morning! Or two. Or four. Dammit, I had four of them, and they were damn good!" I continued vehemently. "Although I could barely re-zip the side of my pants when I was done, it was worth every unhealthy bite. So, don't even attempt to question or judge my choices when my awfully awful breakfast was your everyday meal only months ago. I can't quite do what you're so successfully doing right now, Little Miss Healthy Pants, and I won't have my face rubbed in it," I fumed with no intentions to explain where my entire outburst had come from or whether it would come back soon.

"Little Miss Healthy Pants?" Kristina retorted with a shocked expression completely void of her signature smile. "So, we're not only being ridiculously sarcastic and cruel today, we're also name-calling? That's just great."

"I'm not being sarcastic on this one, Kristina. And, I don't think it's cruel. It's just a perfect name I have for all of my perfect friends who are doing so perfectly well at living so perfectly healthy, and happy, and fit. I think your progress is so super cute to behold that it deserves a super cute name like Little Miss Healthy Pants," I responded with a sarcastic smile, removing every bit of smiling left within her.

"With all due respect that's left to give you right now, Whitney, you and I know there's nothing cute or remotely funny about your rude reasoning behind that name. And, the fact you're being so sarcastic and downright hurtful to me is bewildering. I've been incredibly open with you about how challenging and completely imperfect this entire journey has been for me. Every single pound I've dropped and am finally learning how to keep off has been a struggle to success," Kristina declared as she placed her book back into her tote and turned to walk out of my office. "I won't let your sarcasm, ridicule, and obvious envy steal one bit of my happiness. Nor will I allow your behavior to interrupt my focus in continuing to become completely healthy and fit. I'll take my book and my excitement, and I'll continue moving right along with my goals."

"Kristina, I didn't mean to make you blow a fuse by sarcastically conveying to you that I'm close to blowing my own fuse," I gave her a faint smile, trying to calm us both down a bit.

"Oh, I'm not nearly as angry as you'd like me to be, Whitney. And, I won't be making you angry anymore by wasting your time with a subject that clearly doesn't interest you," she shot back, standing in the door preparing to head down the hall into her office. "However, if and when you decide to stop feeling sorry for yourself as you collect every excuse of why you can't take charge of your life while ridiculing anyone who seems to walk in the courage you won't utilize, just let me know. I'll still choose to be a friend because I really think you're a pretty neat person beyond all your self-hate and sinister comments. Whitney, you clearly know I've been there. I've lived that. I know how tough it is to fight to really get your life and health back. So, if choosing to try to be an inspiration to any willing ear makes me a 'Little Miss Healthy Pants', just tell me where to find the logo. I may have it tattooed on my bikini line, as soon as I find myself a perfect swimsuit at Osh Kosh b' Gosh!" She finished as she marched out with seemingly tear-filled eyes.

"Osh Kosh b' Gosh! Did I say that?" I called after Kristina who was already halfway down the hall as I chuckled in embarrassment and shock, trying to process the sure-fire words she'd hurled at me.

I'd never seen that side of Kristina's mostly beaming personality, nor had I seen such humiliation in her bright blue eyes. The awful feeling in my soul confirming my behavior had indeed hurt her felt absolutely terrible. I sat in complete shame of what a few foul minutes of wallowing in envy and self-pity had possibly done to our friendship.

Kristina had been nothing short of a supportive colleague and an encouraging friend to me from my first interview day at Radiant Reveals. Furthermore, the continued weight loss success she established in her 5 foot 7 inch frame was a constant reminder that my excuses about pursuing my fitness goals were simply excuses. I uncomfortably observed her inside out consistency while raising a 10-year-old autistic child fairly solo as her husband's schedule at the IT firm he owned kept him busy enough to avoid the stress of coping with the needs of their son and the reality of what their marriage had become through years of ignoring it all. Through every bit of her personal chaos she kept her cool, and she kept the encouragement going for herself and so many others, with an overwhelming spirit of gratitude reminding her of how good life really was to her in spite of her life's details.

Kristina shared with me that she had begun to get serious about getting healthy and fit again before her 35th birthday, realizing it'd been over 10 years since she recalled paying any attention to her body at all or being comfortable in her porcelain skin. Having carried more than 235 pounds on her 5'7" frame for years, I completely understood her excitement for losing 70 pounds and counting.

Albeit, the happiness I felt for Kristina drowned in the sea of despair I bore in my own frame. The effects of my weight looked even more repulsive in person than it did on every medical evaluation I'd stared at over the past year alone. I received warning after warning of what was to come if I didn't do the work to eradicate every rampant roll off of my body. Outside my every fear and frustration, the question I contemplated beyond every answer I simply didn't have was how. How would I do what I'd never been able to do? How would I discover how to take control of all that controlled my weight? How would I stop pondering upon how and simply get going as I completely figured out how?

Nonetheless, as much as I wanted to continue dwelling on my frustrating thoughts of despair for a few more moments, I needed to focus on how to muster up an apology that would actually matter to Kristina. Of course I'd have to be figure it out after clearing my morning client roster and heading to lunch with Barb to iron out the details of her spring event coming up way too soon. Hopefully by then, Kristina will have somehow understood that my urge to be a cynical bitch in the face of insecurity proved to be as real as my temptation to eat an entire package of Oreos on a random evening of daydreaming down bad memories lane.

"Sorry I'm a few minutes late. My last morning patient was on full chatterbox mode today. She's finally seeing the results of her laser treatment work just as I promised her she would when she was in full freak out mode weeks ago," I explained to Barb as I plopped down at the tiny table while she smiled a hello to me.

La Jolla's was a quaint deli with a warm aura grander than its blends of eclectic furniture. Their ornamental framed menus displayed a vast list of savory sandwiches and wraps in a manner honoring a rich love for food, fellowship, and good flavors. Barb and I loved the contemporary Old World décor in every detail of the space almost as much as we loved their delectable desserts.

"That's totally okay. I'm just enjoying the ambiance and gathering my thoughts before we start hashing out the details," she responded with her energetic smile. "So, it sounds like things are going fairly well with Dr. Thomas and the gang," she looked at me eagerly, awaiting me to fill her in with every current detail.

"Well, all's okay, overall. My work is really being respected and appreciated, but I'm not quite sure I'm the favorite of the entire gang at the moment after my behavior during a chit-chat this morning," I responded candidly.

"Oh no! Was it another ordeal with a patient who's only *okay* with you while missing Carol's methods?" Barb probed with her sisterly concern.

"Actually, it wasn't a patient at all. It was my colleague, Kristina," I confessed reluctantly.

"Kristina!" Barb exclaimed with her usual naive response of shock to bad news. "I thought she was so great to you so far? What's gotten into her? What in the..."

"It wasn't totally her," I interrupted. "It was me actually. I've just become a bit exhausted with constantly hearing about her weight loss journey and getting loads of far too wonderful advice and encouragement she apparently thinks I need like my next breath. I wasn't entirely mean to her. I just sort of snapped sarcastically and hurt her happy, sensitive feelings," I finished matter-of-factly.

"Whit, are you kidding? As far as I know, from your own words, she's been nothing but tremendously kind and completely supportive to you from the day you interviewed with Radiant Reveals, and now..." She attempted to gather her thoughts in bewilderment.

"Now what, Barb?" I revved up sarcastically. "Now you have something else to judge me on? Barb-1. Whit-0. Let's do lunch!"

"Whit, don't even go there. I'm not judging you, and I'm definitely not trying to smear your face in a mistake because we all make them. Large and small. But just the way you explained how you '*hurt her happy, sensitive feelings*' is filled with the sarcasm I'm sure you spewed all over that conversation or confrontation, or whatever it ended up being. I just don't understand how..." She attempted to finish her lecture on loving-kindness, until I blurted back in.

"You don't understand how what? How perfect you are, yet how those apples seemed to rot on

73

every branch of my side of the family tree?" I hissed. "Oh, no. You do rub it in Barb. You also make sure it sinks in during most every conversation or stupid lunch we attempt to have."

"Are we really going to start this drama again, Whit? Really? After we just made amends weeks ago. As I sit here seriously agonizing a bit on how to curtail around the reality that you've probably already arrived here a bit frustrated about the fact you're not consistently working towards the fitness goals you wanted to achieve before this event," she retorted in a tone filled with anxiety.

"Oh don't curtail around anything, Barb. Just say what your judgmental mind hides so well behind your sweet, sisterly smile. *'I can't believe I have such a fat ass as a cousin and a best friend. I can't believe after all these years of giving her so much of my amazing advice and superb support that she still hasn't come even close to reaching her goals. And, I can't understand how in my being such an example of what perfection really is, it hasn't somehow rubbed off on her by now,'*" I hissed as I mocked the words I was sure she'd always thought about me.

"Oh my God! Seriously? Do you seriously think I look down on you, and detest you, and think of you in any of the negative ways you choose to think and talk about yourself? What's wrong with you, Whit?" Barb exclaimed in full-blown annoyance.

"You're actually part of what's wrong with me, Barbie!" I shot back as I shrugged my shoulders, preparing to completely unleash what was left of my

74

frustrated energy upon her. "You've been a pain in my fat ass ever since I can remember, parading your bony ass around with your perfect positive energy and every other facet of your perfectly perfect life. Perfect grades in school. Perfect body damn near out of the womb. Perfect husband who's the only other person in your world as nearly perfect as you. Perfect kids, in a pair even," I recalled her twin boys, Ethan and Evan, who were just as charming and gorgeous as she and Rick were. "Little Miss Healthy Pants has it all," I finished with what I was sure was a fire breathed snarl.

Barb's 7-year-old boys not only had her gorgeous husband Rick's wavy, sun-kissed dirty blonde hair but they also donned his grayish blue eyes and seemed all set to grow as tall as their 6-foot 4 inch dad as their baby boyish faces were adorably misplaced on their already five foot tall frames. Even at 35 years of age, Rick was a keen replica of the hottie underwear model we all wish to take home but are happy just to gawk at in our favorite magazine. Though he'd actually done a few modeling jobs for fun before entering law school, he moved on to pursue his family's career heritage of law and politics, becoming a prominent attorney in North Dallas with his uncle's firm and eventually being selected as an Assistant District Attorney in Greater Dallas. Rick could easily be mistaken for a typical pretty boy at first glance, yet moments upon meeting him, one could gather and agree he was one to hold his own in most any setting despite his almost too good-looking for a guy appearance.

From the time they began dating in high school as a freshman cheerleader and a senior football captain, Barb tried her best to portray Rick and herself as a normal couple. Though their eventual marriage solidified their status as a prominent and powerful extension of his already well-known Dallas family, she was amazing at portraying their household as refreshingly modest amongst their marvelous perks and possessions. It was one of her several motives in why she hosted an annual spring event for charity orchestrated on their expansive lawn in their gated community inhabited by several of the who's who in Dallas and American society. Barb was also undeniably admirable in how she kept a solid hand in raising their two boys amidst their hired help while balancing the responsibilities of Rick's hectic public schedule and her swanky duties as a full-time socialite. Their lives were consumed by far too many beautiful and important people who couldn't get enough of the beauty of the both of them and the influence they held in an extremely influential city as Dallas.

"Oh. My. God. I'm not your problem, Whit," Barb responded as she shook her head with a methodical calm I somewhat sensed was the set up for quite a storm. "You are your own problem. Not even the weight you've grown to despise is your ultimate problem. *You* are your problem. It's so disappointing to know you seriously cannot see that, but here goes," she continued on far too calmly. "I do see clearly now that it hasn't served either of us well for me to continue on trying to tone down who I am in order to accommodate your insecurity and absurd jealously. Yes, I have long and lean legs. Yes, I have lean and toned arms. Yes, I have a firm ass and a flat stomach. And yes, I've consistently worked hard to maintain all of that, but not nearly as much as I've labored to develop a positive mental attitude and a solid heart—both of which are so full of positive energy and compassion. I truly don't have the desire to spew at you a well-deserved counterattack of even half of the hateful words, comments, and hilariously unfunny jokes you've thrown at me. Every comment concerning my weight or lack of weight as long as I can remember or can..."

"Argh! You are such a..." I interrupted before Barb interjected again with a seriously abrupt tone.

"Such a what, Whit? A ridiculous rail? A boisterous beanpole? A skinny bitch? What other lame and callous name are you ready to hurl at me?" She stared back at me with a precarious steadiness in her voice. "I've finally had more than enough of your ratchet behavior and ridicule wrapped in self-pity as you piss on every bit of support most anyone tries to offer you. I seriously don't know what's it going to take for you to realize that tossing all of your hate and hurtful words at me won't take one single pound off of your body or soothe the misery in your soul. Focusing on who you think I shouldn't be or what you think I shouldn't have will never help you attain anything you really want or cause you to become who you really desire to be," she continued with a compassionate yet fire-breathing intensity I hadn't quite seen in her, ever. "And Whit, please know I don't fret about any of the weight you've gained over time, or the weight you haven't lost. Do you know what I actually agonize about concerning you?" She paused, choking back tears that caused her bright brown eyes to glisten. "I actually rack my brain about how you still haven't grasped the reality of how strong, and powerful, and beautiful you are because you're so damned focused on constantly attacking any beauty or strength you think is so tremendous in anyone else—anyone who rubs your insecurity the wrong way. While I seriously can't wait to one day celebrate you losing the weight that's robbed you of so much health and happiness, I look forward much more to seeing you get rid of the lack of confidence in you. It's robbed you of way too much, including your sanity at times. I just…"

"Barb, I can't believe you're taking this…" I attempted to interrupt again before she shot a solemn look at me conveying the message of *shut up and don't speak until motioned*.

"Whit, it's your choice to continue to pout around in your own darkness and despair of what you think you can't do and can't be. It's always been *your* choice. You know my life. You know that nothing about it has ever been perfect—inside or outside of the gym in my '*she's so perfect*' body.

Need I remind you that the same stares and glares you feel like you're always getting, I also deal with my own brand of them on a daily basis?" She continued on with as much empathy as irritation in her voice. "From the brainless bigots amongst Rick's network of the rich and ridiculous who consider it a bit vexing to encounter an attractive bi-racial woman with actual brains in tow. To the ill-mannered haters at the gym who stare and whisper loosely about me during my workouts as if I'm somehow overstaying my welcome because I'm fairly fit. The idiots have no idea that the issues of my mitral valve prolapse heart condition doesn't allow me to do the half of what I'd really like to do in my workout time," she continued on as the dam of her every frustration broke freely. "Let's not start on the countless women I've trained myself to smile a genuine smile towards even through their menacing glances spewing envy and disgust at the sight of another 'skinny bitch' like me garnering the attention of a man who's attention they apparently aren't keeping—an ogling issue that has nothing to do with me, or them for that matter. I fully know that because I've been on the receiving end of having my man step beyond our bedroom to have his desires fulfilled elsewhere despite who he has in life and in his bed," she lectured on with a fire burning much deeper than the words I'd ever torched her with. "I don't have any hate to give to you, Whit, or anyone else, because I know how horrid it feels to be on the receiving end of it. Perfect has never been in my DNA or ingrained in my life's details, although the pain of being hated for seeming to be perfect while enjoying a seemingly perfect life has. Even now as I deal with the continued craziness of Rick's career and Dad's way too public legal challenges, you know how tough it's been for me to deal. It's been tough to deal with all of it. You know that. But, you know what? You also need to know that this is the day I'm choosing to never again be mistreated or disrespected by you simply because you won't take the time to tap into your own self-worth. I won't do it anymore," she stood up abruptly with a sincere yet strained smile.

"Where are you going? We haven't gone over the event schedule yet," I asked as I barely looked up at her in complete embarrassment.

"We both know it wouldn't be wise to continue on this afternoon. And no, I'm not angry at you. I'm completely angry at myself for taking this crap from you for far too long," she finished with the same boldness I'd seen in her when she confronted Uncle Steve a couple of months before concerning the last DUI almost landing him in prison. "I'll simply email you the final details about everything later this evening. I do hope to see you there. It'll be a great time."

"Ok, so I'll just..." I halted my response as Barb walked out briskly with a wave over her shoulder to confirm our conversation was virtually over.

CHAPTER FIVE

Yes, it's hard!

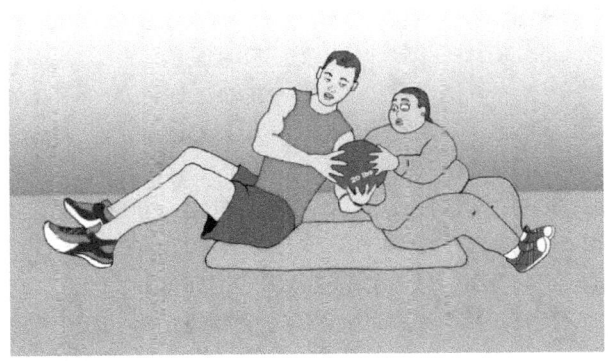

"Two rows of Oreos and a half quart of the best mint chocolate chip ice cream later, and I still sat in frustration beyond words, pondering on all the exhausting words I'd exchanged with Kristina, and with Barb. My heated exchanges with damn near everyone came to mind, as I reflected back on the past year alone of the roller-coaster of emotions I'd endured in attempt to do everything yet much of nothing concerning my weight.

The reality wrecking me wasn't only the fact that they were mostly right as I was wrong, but it was in also realizing I'd been off my rocker for so long. Even in my junk food induced stupor, I looked back at how Julian had been dead-on concerning much about me. Somewhere in the midst of packing on the extra pounds and throwing away every bit of confidence to lose it, I'd become a version of myself I could no longer tolerate. I could no longer conceal my own personal despair in my everyday words, choices and behavior. I absolutely hated being so cruel to Barb, yet I hated more what I looked and felt like in the more than 250 pounds on my 5'4" frame. It was tougher than anything to understand why I no longer tried my damnedest to be pleasant to most anyone who was a constant reminder of who I was and who I'd probably never be as I just couldn't seem to get my ass in gear and do something, or anything, about the weight I was far too miserable about. Even as I eventually coughed up an apology to Kristina, mentioning my catastrophic lunch with Barb, I was ridiculously honest in admitting to her that if she didn't possess such a positive attitude about her weight loss journey, it probably wouldn't be such an irritation to me. Yet, her positivity infused me with actual hope during many days I'd considered quitting on aspects of life itself much less my many attempts at pursuing my fitness goals.

My physique had been larger than my delicious smoked Christmas ham display as long as I could remember. I'd already crept past 250 pounds with the frightening reality of another plateau of pounds waiting just around the corner on the scale. I couldn't deal anymore. I'd tried it all, and I'd quit it all. I'd broken more promises to myself than I could recall. I'd burned bridge after bridge to most every road of help and advice offered to me. The reminders of my frustrating flops and failures were everywhere around me.

Stacks of fitness DVDs which I barely viewed much less completed lay overlooked amongst my library of home movies. My kitchen counter was filled with hardly used health food cookbooks, along with miracle diet manuals and planners. I had folders of every color stuffed with magazine tear outs of revolutionary at home work-outs. Trendy workout apps were downloaded on my phone along with various celebrity work-outs programs. Expensive pieces of workout equipment, along with other must have fitness gadgets, lay forgotten in a spare bedroom once considered my motivational home gym. Its use was as welcomed as a plate of grilled chicken and asparagus on a long awaited a cheat day.

The evidence was clear. I'd tried again and again without triumph. I had started over and over without staying the course. Even more, I often quit faster than the time it took me to muster up the courage to actually begin at all. To try to explain to my 11-year-old Emily why I was always too exhausted to function or attend numerous functions with her was more unbearable than constantly trying to find decent clothing to cover up my ever expanding size 20 frame.

There was a part of me considering walking the five miles or so to the gym, especially as my car oftentimes tended to veer off to a fast food place instead of directly to Dynamo Fitness. I was contemplating marching up to that hottie of a trainer, Cory, and declaring to him to do whatever he wanted with my body, transformation first. Nonetheless, the other part of me felt far more courageous and comfortable in continuing on in my stupor of eating, gaining, and complaining. It always seemed to hurt less than the process of getting back into the process of determining to be fit all over again.

"Mom?" Emily startled the bejesus out of me, calling out while walking towards the kitchen. I hadn't expected her home for another hour, considering Tracy always took her sweet time on her designated carpool day for the girls' after school pickup at the Y.

"Hi sweetheart! You're home early today," I replied, scrambling to grab a paper towel to wipe the crumbs I could feel all over my face.

I internally freaked out knowing what Emily would probably say or think at the display of the package of ransacked Oreos and half slaughtered quart of ice cream sprawled out on the kitchen island next to the bag of chips I'd just ripped into moments before she walked in. I'd promised her the weekend before I'd be starting a new diet on Monday in efforts to probably, I'd emphasized probably, join her in the Mom & Me Fun Run race being hosted by the Y in the next month or so. She'd excitedly told me about it the day they announced it, and I had yet to give her persistent questioning a solid answer. She desperately wanted to be a part of what all of her friends were apparently doing, and the thought of being the mom who ruined it for her sent me reeling at every mention of it.

"Dad picked me up from afterschool today because he wanted to talk to me about something important," she responded, giving me the *Mom, I really hope you're listening to me'* look.

Although Emily had her dad's stunning dark eyes, delicate lips, and perfectly pointed yet well-rounded nose, she was growing up, or rather growing out, to have my physique. She was a heart wrenching reflection of the weight issues I endured at her age, and she was completely aware of it at only 11 years old. She was already concerned that her beautiful long brown hair wasn't doing a wonderful job of hiding the rolls developing around her torso as she carried 140 pounds on her 5'1" frame. I knew I should do even more to consistently steer her well in her nutrition, yet it was already tough to deal in my own frustrating frame without dealing with the aggravation of Julian's questioning about the health habits I was and wasn't teaching her. While I would be the first to admit we didn't eat as perfect as he and his psycho pseudo-Barbie girlfriend, Karen, I was definitely a parent who made sure Emily ate more fruit and veggies than I could personally tolerate, drank lots of water, and rested well with a bedtime void of computers or late-night TV.

Being that she possessed the strong persona of a college student simply visiting a middle school, she hadn't had to weather the bullying we knew could come with living in a heavier frame at her snobbish prep school. In fact, Emily had been the umpire in several incidents of bullying and unnecessary teasing. Her solid blend of charm, humor, and fearlessness helped her to hold her own pretty well as an 11-year-old. Although her stubborn strength caused us to have to often remind her that Julian and I were the parents and not otherwise, her powerful spirit always made us smile as much as her adorably cute face.

"I'm listening, Emmy. Is he rethinking his career again?" I responded without trying to hide my sarcasm.

As well as Julian did in his investment banking career, he'd always had a passion for fitness. He and Karen seemed to attend and support every 5k run, wellness event, and notable gym opening announced in Dallas. The more he committed himself to chiseling away at his own body, the more he seemed to convince himself he should be helping others to do the same. His perfect swolemate [the nickname he and Karen often called each other, making Emily laugh while I literally hurled on the inside] was a shining example of his apparent expertise while my huge ass had been his hugest flop. I loved to remind myself that Julian wasn't as awesome as he thought he was, even at the expense of having to admit I was even more enormous and enormously out of shape as when he and I officially parted ways.

"No, he actually asked Miss Karen to marry him. They're engaged, and they're getting married in Hawaii. He wants me to be a part of the ceremony.

It's during Thanksgiving, so he said he knew it would be a big deal to let everyone know in advance," she explained while glancing away uncomfortably as she did when she knew I most likely wouldn't be responding with a smile.

"Oh, how great. So, he thought interrupting your afterschool program time was the best way to share such good news?" I responded without trying to hide my frustration or resentment for such an announcement. I knew the day would come. I also knew it would come on a day when I just couldn't handle hearing any more bad news or good news equally as bad as bad news.

"I knew you wouldn't be okay with it, Mom. Dad said he wanted me to be the first to know, and he'd get with you about all the details soon. I didn't want you to be totally surprised by it," she shared in hopes her explanation would help the situation a bit.

"I'm okay, Emmy. I knew this day would be coming for them soon. I'm actually happy for them. It should be really neat to chat with him about it all." I lied, seriously swallowing down the flood of tears bubbling through every part of my soul.

Even though it had been three full years since our divorce, it still ached as much as it did from the first day of our separation to lose the only man I had ever truly loved, even when I hadn't had much love for myself. Julian and I were inseparable from the start, until I somehow allowed an awful blend of pride and insecurity, as explained by my therapist, to primarily control me and ultimately separate us. Although I thought it was my love for all things food

87

that caused us to crumble, it was mostly my resistance to his resistance of my destructive choices. It would ultimately take our marriage to the curb of divorce and leave me to lament on the curb of despair. As much as I longed to fix everything I knew was breaking our marriage, I had no energy to fight for myself nor for us anymore. Nonetheless, I fought to the bitter end to convey that all of our problems hadn't been solely due to my problems.

Even as I looked around at the rustic glam décor of the spacious two-story home Emily and I lived in as our new version of family, I couldn't always wrap my ahead around the fact that Julian would never walk through the enormous front door after a long day as my exhausted husband to greet me with a hello or ignore my greetings of to-do's or complaints. He'd never again lie in bed next to me with passion to enjoy every part of me, or tossing about with words of full-blown frustration as I demanded he crash on the couch because of everything and nothing. He'd never again be in the driver's seat of either of our luxury vehicles turning up the radio to drown out a silly argument, or worse, standing outside of the bathroom door shouting as I threatened to drown him in the tub for rushing me yet again when he knew that late is how I function. Our version of marriage was over. Even more, as the ass I often told him to kiss in frustration continued to expand, hopes of my ever marrying again seemed to be nearing game over.

"So, I know this probably isn't the best time, but can you inform me now about whether you're doing the Fun Run with me?" Emily interrupted my daydreaming down memory lane again with her grown up voice she'd been working on as one of her New Year's resolutions. "They made a few more cool announcements about it today, and I have to reserve our spot for the early bird rate by Friday. I don't want to be the last kid to register us to do it, Mom."

"We haven't discussed how you actually feel about Dad's news yet, and you're already chalking out my to-do list for the week," I muttered while trying to figure out how to end the long line of questioning I knew was stirring in my persistent child about my participation in that God forbidden event. "I'm still not sure, Emmy. I don't want to commit to do something I may have to back out of later, disappointing you even more. We're much busier at the office when spring is approaching because almost everyone in Dallas is getting ready to change from winter to pre-summer skin. I'd rather use those weekends for rejuvenating instead of running about doing everything. You know that."

"So, what you're telling me is I can just forget about it like you forgot about your diet this week?" Emily responded with a snarky tone, scanning the kitchen island still cluttered with a few of the fixings from my snack attack.

"Excuse me, young lady. Your tone is as rude as your little pot shot comment. I'm sticking to my diet this week. I simply had a rough day that an 11-year-old brain couldn't even begin to comprehend," I retorted with an embarrassment that couldn't hide my lying to the both of us.

"Mom, I don't mean to be rude, but you told me I should always speak my mind because no one can hear what I'm not saying," she looked directly at me with a helpless defiance. "I just don't get it. You're a doctor. Well, almost a doctor. We don't really do anything healthy people do. I'd ask Dad to do the run with me, but he's not my mom; he's my dad. I won't ask Miss Karen because I know you'd be pissed at me and her."

"Pissed? So you're not only being disrespectful, but you're also using disrespectful language? Emily, what's gotten into you!" I exclaimed in further humiliation with a mixture of shock.

"I don't mean to be disrespectful, Mom. It just sucks that my mom is the only mom who doesn't do anything with me except go to the grocery store or to a new restaurant when it opens. If we ever go to the mall, it's barely for an hour because you don't like to walk around. Even during Christmas, we only walked through one section of the coolest mall in Dallas. You got so tired and annoyed you decided to come home and buy everything else online. Mom, you don't... you don't even get out of the car when you come to pick us up for your carpool day on Fridays. You just sit there while all the other moms..." She ranted on in fully dramatic 11-year-old mode before I interrupted her with my best *I'm the mom* voice, sensing her understandable frustration would cause her to say something that would completely destroy what was left of my fragile emotions from an already emotional day.

"Is there anything else you need to add to your 'My Mom Sucks' list before I blow what's left of my already short fuse today, Emily Marie?" I interjected.

"Mom, I'm not trying to make you feel bad or make you mad at me. I'm just trying to tell you why it sucks so bad to have you say no to the run. You say no to almost everything," she began to pace about the kitchen floor, trying to further explain herself. "I know that when adults think they can't really do something they try to avoid it, but you're not the only mom that's a large mom who's going to do the run. Miss Tracy is large. She's probably larger than all the moms who'll be there, but she and Lexie were like the first people to sign up for it," she wailed on.

She was dead-on about Tracy being big, as she'd probably already passed the 300 pound plateau on the bathroom scale years ago. Tracy was my favorite eat out buddy. She was also one of my only friends to understand that real women have curves and rolls, and we aren't willing to waste time figuring out the difference between the both. She and her husband were still happily together as his frame was even larger than hers. Clark always made us crack up with laughter when he proclaimed that 'Sexy Claus', his nickname for himself, couldn't do life without Mrs. Claus keeping him happy and fed. Tracy and Clark had become my best of friends since Emily and I moved into our neighborhood almost three years ago. They were also my unofficial frenemies [best friends yet worst enemies] during the fleeting moments in time when I decided to get back on the band wagon of getting fit. Their love for all things food always connected to the best and worst of me.

"Well Emmy, I'm not Tracy, and the last time I checked you weren't switched at birth, so you're not Lexie." I shot back with the last ounces of energy I had to continue our bickering. "I told you I'll think about it. Today is Monday. Friday is still days away. And, it's not the very last day to register."

"Don't worry about it, Mom. I'll deal with it. I'm already learning how to deal with my friends who think it's so funny to use you in their 'Your mama's so fat' jokes. Not to mention, they're suggesting I maybe find an agent to help me audition for a kids' version of Weight Watchers commercials," she blurted out in a matter of fact tone I knew was more to detail the frustration of her heart rather than to hurt mine. "I'm going upstairs to start my homework. I'll come back down and grab dinner later."

I didn't dare attempt to call after her as she bounded up the stairs. I stood in a shockwave of silence as my heart broke in shameful realization of the many instances in one day reminding me of what my life was like as opposed to what it really could be. And the open bag of chips staring at me from the kitchen counter couldn't even begin to fix all that was shattered in hearing the words spilled from my child's heart, or dealing with the effects of the ones that had spewed out of my soul throughout the day.

"Yes, it's hard! It'll always be difficult to some degree, Whit. But, you know what's really hard? Living on tons of medication to barely survive because you decided doing what it takes to stay healthy and fit was too hard," Cory continued his fervent preaching to me during our grueling session. "And, waking up completely tired in the morning after you already went to bed exhausted the night before because an inactive body doesn't rest well. That's hard. Or, not fully experiencing a great vacation because your energy level limits you from enjoying or exploring much of anything outside the menu at every restaurant table you plop down to yet can barely get up from. That's hard, and it's unacceptable if you really want to enjoy the details of your life."

"Are you ever going to stop all of your preaching to me?" I sniggered at him with the last of the breath left in me from his 'Do or Die' plank challenge.

I couldn't believe over three weeks had already passed since I mustered up the courage to reach out to Cory and try once again to get my life and body back in working order. I made the move immediately after the day from hell I endured in my eye-opening catfights with Kristina and Barb, followed by the crushing realization that my Emily was suffering at school because I refused to suffer the process of doing what it required to get my body and my health back. The agony my weak muscles and messed up mentality about food and fitness experienced with

Cory often felt unbearable. Nonetheless, it was worth it to see the results of already having to purchase a new size in office wear. I also had real energy during the day for the first time in my adult life since I was a grad student in college.

Cory was as empathetic as his 6-foot 3 inch frame was tall. Yet, he was tougher on me than any of my deep desires to call it quits in the middle of each set of every tough exercise he put my physique through. His programming scheduled me to workout for one relentless hour twice a day, six days a week. Whether I was scheduled to workout with him or workout solo, his specifically guided details were paying off, and the work was always tough as nails. From the never ending squats and suicide runs, to the burpees and battle rope slams, to the plank work and pushup combos, nothing was off limits for him to bring to our workout sessions. And virtually no excuse, outside of death or a collapse before death, was ever acceptable for me to bail out of any facet of our overall program.

"Are you ever going to stop trying to convince me of what you can't do?" He shot back with his signature grin that melted my heart in the smooth voice that made me furious at myself for enjoying it at the most inopportune times. "Whit, with the demand of both our schedules, I've only got one full hour twice a week to be face to face with you and somehow help you grasp the reality that you really can come to a point where you completely understand how to take care of your body well. The fact that I know my main responsibility is to help you recognize that more than 99% of what you accomplish physically will only happen as you become stronger mentally, I've got to let it rip every time I know you're feeling like what we're doing is only meant to rip you to shreds. So, unless you want me to stop our session to grab some fancy cheese to go with your wonderful whine, Princess, let's do this," he finished with a laugh.

"Aye! Aye! Captain Crazy," I shot back sarcastically at him, throwing back my exhausted right arm to toss a silly salute his way. "Can you at least give me credit that I wasn't saying *I can't*, knowing the stance you have about that phrase, and every other phrase that doesn't breed positivity and power?" I teased a bit more. "I was just talking about how hard this crap still is. You'd think after over three straight weeks of all this ass kicking, my body would somehow stop aching through all of it. I'm just wondering if I'll ever actually like this craziness. Like, really like it. Like my crazy cousin Barb does, and like you do," I tried to explain in full exhaust mode, hoping we were near cool down or that my attempt at another chit-chat would push the time on to cool down mode.

"I'd think after three weeks of dropping 18 pounds and 5 inches from your waist that you'd be a bit happier in your tone, yet it's still as whiney as a teething baby," he laughed while giving me the same mocking look he'd given when I asked him whether or not it was okay to grab fast food for breakfast after our last training session. "I've told you before, Whit, it doesn't ever really become easy breezy when we choose to workout effectively. Our body does get better and stronger at the process of getting through it though. I know you think I breeze through everything, but my personal workouts still slaughter me. I'm able to push through all of it because of the power in my muscles and my mind to endure it now. Just the fact you now have the courage and actual stamina to do that mile and a half fun run with your daughter in a couple of weeks should tell you everything about what this crazy stuff can really start to feel like," he smiled in complete admiration of me.

Cory was so right. In the few weeks of seriously taking heed to everything he had instructed me to do, it was working as effectively as my muscles were sore. From adding vegetables to literally every meal I ate, to getting rid of my beloved pastries, sodas, and lattes I never thought would leave my psyche, I hadn't only dropped 18 pounds and 5 inches but I also gained more confidence than I even knew was in me. My conversations at work had begun to pour with positivity as I felt so much better about myself than I ever imagined possible just a month before. Just the thought of being able to do so many exercises I'd convinced myself a heavy body like mine could never do was unbelievable as I somehow developed so much strength and persistence to complete every set of everything Cory consistently preached me through. To be able to keep my word to Emily and be fully prepared to complete that 1 and ½ mile Fun Run meant more to me than any favorite comfort food I was daily deciding to say a resounding 'Hell no' to.

"You're right. If I'd known your craziness would have me losing weight like Santa Claus captured at a veggie farm, I would've let you start murdering me on the day we first chatted after that elliptical almost killed me," I laughed with a sense of pride in who I'd already become in comparison to the impudent woman my genius trainer had met during one of the worst, yet luckiest days of my life.

Cory had not only become an amazing strength and support to me, but we also got along in a way that made me look forward to every grueling session and left me smiling through every bead of sweat that covered me afterwards. The way he saw completely through me and still seemed to accept and understand every broken part of me meant even more than the amazing tips and insight he constantly poured out to me.

"Ha-ha! Well, we're not even halfway through your initial phase of training, so hopefully you're still Team Cory through the next levels of torture I have in store for you," he teased with a seriousness he could never quite hide from his playful voice. "Like I told you from our first session together Whit, I'll always be excited with you about the weight you continue to lose, but the ultimate goal is for you to gain insight and confidence on how to do fit and healthy as a lifestyle so that the extra weight and all the issues surrounding it won't be your nemesis anymore. The scale is important. The size we carry is important. However, it's nothing in comparison to the health profile that steps on a scale, or the energy and stamina that struts around in whatever size you are."

"You and that insight of yours! I bet you really do sleep with The Science Channel on, don't you?" I teased him with admiration of the expertise and encouragement he always loaded me with.

"No. I actually sleep with a night-light on and a specific warning alarm for the days I'm training with Princess Whitney Cordona!" He laughed out loud at the response on my face.

"Ha-ha! If I had any feeling left in my arms, I'd knuckle sandwich you, Coach Crazy! You already know we big girls don't cry; we bite," I made him laugh out loud once again at my self-deprecating joke that was always funnier said than actually lived.

"Whit, you barely reach my kneecaps on a really good day, so I'm not much worried about you tackling me," he playfully pushed at my shoulder while laughing even harder at the fact that I was so much shorter than him.

"Yes, I'm vertically challenged, but you're talking a lot of noise, my friend. My squat strength alone should remind you of the capabilities in this short and sexy frame," I shot back with a facetious laugh, making no attempt to hide my flirtation.

"Yeah, you're bringing sexy back, but that won't stop me from making you pay for your knuckle sandwich threat with a good elbow hug to the jaw," he laughed as he hilariously demonstrated the attack while dancing aimlessly over my short stature. "If you weren't a dear client of mine, I'd land this elbow on top of your tiny head," he laughed even harder.

"How did this dear client ever come about trusting such a crazy person to get me in shape?" I laughed even more at the bantering back and forth between us.

"Because you're much smarter than your heart is able to understand at the moment, Princess Whit," he replied with a smirk that said everything I could only hope he could be possibly thinking about the growing friendship in our sessions together.

CHAPTER SIX

Hate My Life Without You?

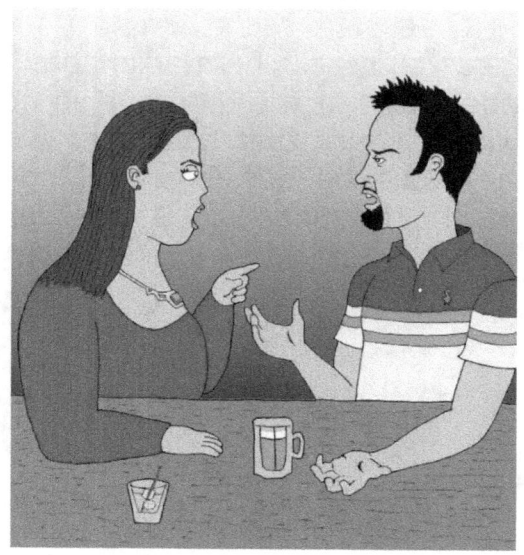

"So, what's the big deal about Emmy staying for the entire trip to Hawaii for the wedding, Whit?" Julian probed, staring at me intently with his piercing brown eyes. After all the years we'd been apart, his features were still a bit breathtaking to me although I often wanted to knock the breath completely out of him almost every time we were forced to have another necessary parental chit-chat. Yet, even in the toughest of conversations, it was tough to ignore the powerful combo of his bronzed olive skin, dark hair, piercing brown eyes, and delicate lips projecting every word from his deep Latino voice.

From the day I responded to the initial greeting of his 6-foot 2 inch frame, it was clear that Julian was one of the toughest versions of a pretty boy I'd ever come across. We met during our personal workout time at Baylor University's student life center almost immediately after we'd both started our grad school programs. It was love at first lunge when he felt the need to offer me 'good insight' concerning my balance and form as I struggled across the free weight area in attempts to build a firm ass and get rid of the flab my thighs had collected during the four years of food and fiestas incorporated into undergrad life.

By the time our workout session was over, nothing mattered inside of that distinctive gym outside of the intriguing crush he and I seemed to have almost immediately on each other. The energy we shared in our first conversation became the foundation of the friendship and fiery romance we built straightway. We laughed and flirted and worked harder than we ever would've worked during what would've been a typical Thursday night at the gym.

Two and a half years later, we were excitedly married after not being able to hold off on an unofficial engagement or an official pregnancy before graduation. Though my physique grew farther and farther from the woman he'd first met, I was incredibly thankful to still have a hot husband. I was even more thankful our darling Emily took on so much of his dark Latino features. My own DNA strands of having a White mom and a Latino dad somehow only took on my mom's green eyes and dark brown hair while my Dad's golden Latino complexion apparently went to my brother to enjoy.

"Julian, I know you're totally excited about finally marrying Karen, but the bigger deal is the fact that Emmy isn't nearly as thrilled about the nuptials as we'd all hope for," I responded, trying my best to take the diplomatic approach in what I sensed would be a tough conversation. "Because she's so in love with her daddy, she just doesn't know how to tell you that she's not in love with watching you marry Karen. So, I believe if we force her to be there the entire 10 days versus just doing a long weekend for it, it'll be a bigger deal for all of us. Emmy's mature for her age, but she's still just a kid. She's a kid preparing to watch her dad officially and completely build another family, when all she's ever known is our version of family that ended barely three years ago," I continued in full effort to help him understand our ordeal really wasn't just about he and Karen's great day.

"Yes, it was barely three years ago. Whit, you and I know our version of family was mostly over by the time Emmy was three years old. I'm sure you've even looked back and wondered as I have on how we were even able to actually push on for another five years," he replied matter-of-factly yet with a carefulness I didn't quite recognize. "I just hope this doesn't have anything to do with your not liking this, or not liking Karen."

"Ha-ha!" I laughed out loud at his asinine response. "Julian, it doesn't matter whether I like you getting remarried or not. Emmy is who matters right now. And what's there to like about Karen? She's a two-faced, conniving cheater whose narcissism runs as deep as the Grand Canyon. Like I told you before in our previous chat when I officially congratulated you on your engagement, you two really deserve one another. So, congratulations, again. I really do wish you both the best," I continued on with a little more emotion than I was planning to bring to our discussion. "I also wish you and I can agree that the best way to ensure Emmy will be her best self in all of this is by simply having her spend that weekend in Hawaii with you and Karen. She'll still be able to take part in your actual wedding, and I'm sure she won't miss all of your nuptial festivities. She can fly out early Thursday morning, and it's totally okay that she returns later on Monday and is back to school that following Wednesday. She can rest up on Tuesday, if needed, from the time change of the trip.

"Seriously? Thursday is still Thanksgiving Day on the calendar, Whit!" He snarled at me.

"I'm aware of that, Julian, and you and I are both aware it's the least busy day to fly during the Thanksgiving holiday season. It's not an easy call, but it should work. I'm already sacrificing having a decent Thanksgiving break with her, as you're scheduled to have her for Christmas this year. I'm sure you can find it in your understanding heart to sacrifice your need to bellyache about her not being in Hawaii hand in hand with you and Karen for 10 days," I hissed back as my mama bear instincts rose even higher.

"Aye! I thought you'd become a bit nicer as you've dropped all this weight. Don't you even feel nicer?" He laughed while trying to diffuse what we both knew could be an incredibly awful argument. "You are looking great by the way, and you seem far more energetic. The fact that you participated in the Fun Run with Emmy is huge. She's still through the moon about it, and she said you did better than so many other moms out there."

"Thank you. I have a really amazing trainer who seems to be great at helping me understand that I'm really as great as I choose to be. Over the past two months I've dropped about 40 pounds and lost 8 inches, and I'm 3 sizes smaller," I smiled with a confidence that had certainly not been there months before. "The run was a bit challenging at first, but it was actually fun. It was pretty amazing to be able to do something like that with Emmy and not absolutely die or cause her to die of embarrassment," I finished with a proud chuckle.

"Wow. That's awesome! Who would have thought that...," Julian exclaimed with a smile.

"Yeah, who would have thought?" I interrupted him quickly for fear he would remind me of the days

104

he and I knew weren't the best of times: the days I had no motivation to get out of bed, much less complete a mile and a half run. "Speaking of change, you must admit I've been rather n ce in all of this. In fact, if I hadn't decided early on to be kind in my dealings with your wonderful engagement, Karen would've already gotten a huge box of black congratulations roses from me weeks ago," I laughed out loud at the thought of something like that coming to my mind, much less coming out of my mouth.

"Aye! You are bitter. Black roses? In a huge box?" He laughed heartily while looking away uneasily from our spot at the bar as we both seemed to realize we hadn't shared real laughter in a conversation in quite some time.

Having a strong drink at a swanky bar was often the only way Julian and I could get through a significant parental chat without being tempted to toss the contents of the entire room at each other, much less a few rude words. The upscale atmosphere of Emery's had just enough ambiance to make us feel a bit calmer in each other's presence and just enough attendance of influential patrons to keep us well behaved if the details of our conversation caused us to want to co ludicrous. Plus, the seating in Emery's Art Deco themed space wasn't too cute for comfort, and guests were never made to feel uncomfortable in casual attire.

"I'm not bitter, at least not as much as I used to be," I admitted with a half-smile. "It's tough at times watching Emmy grow up and emulate so much of who you are. It's also hard not to wonder in regret of how good things could've been between us today if you and Karen hadn't decided to fall head over heels for each other as everyone else's heads were knocked off in the process."

"Whit, I don't want to rehash the past, but let's be real. If things had been so good between us, Karen wouldn't have ever happened. She wouldn't have happened at all," he responded with conviction. "The last thing I ever imagined doing in life was cheating on the woman I loved and built a life and a family with, but..."

"But, I got fat, and Mr. Amazing with his amazing muscles and relentless motivation to have a perfect wife again couldn't sustain himself around a fabulously fit femme fatale who was simply looking for another opportunity to shop for a living," I interrupted, tossing all efforts to hide what was still left of my bitterness. "How's her new couture blog going anyway? It really is a great career choice for her."

"Whit, do we really want to go down this road again? I've said I'm sorry more times than I can remember. My only relentless behavior has been in making sure our beautiful Emmy knows that our divorce was never about her, and none of the decisions surrounding it will ever change how much we both love her," he continued in an exhausted tone. "I can't change the past, and if you want to rehash, it be prepared to at least tell the entire truth about it. You hadn't allowed me to really touch you for years before Karen came on the scene. Even before that, the few times we had any intimate interaction was after rounds of pleading with you and then rounds of apologies afterwards for bothering you at all because of how you felt about your body," he finished just as his voice rose to fume mode.

"So, it was all me," I responded with the air of humiliation about our split-up that just didn't seem to go away. "Julian was the perfect husband who was just abused and ignored."

"I never said it was all you, Whit, and I never will. You constantly barraging me and making me out to be an uncontrollable, cheating asshole certainly isn't true. Your version of that lame story has gotten old," he responded in exasperation, pressing his hands into the mahogany bar counter. "Whit, I did everything I thought I could do to repair our marriage. No matter what I did, it was never enough. Even if it was seemingly enough, it was never understood. I didn't hold you to any outrageous standards of keeping a perfect body. I understood you had birthed our beautiful girl. Hell, I even wanted us to have more kids. Yet, the more you decided to choose not to do anything consistently about your weight or health, the more it wrecked the desire for anything and everything else we both wanted."

"Your trying was your relentless nit-picking that just never let up, Julian. I tried to stick to eating your exhausting lists of everything healthy. I seriously tried to stay on-board with your extreme workout schedule while raising an animated kid who mirrors your stubbornness and energy level. All of that on top of building a career that's never been very easy, although it's been completely rewarding. You just didn't seem to understand that I was your wife and not your clone," I fumed back at him with full resentment. "I wasn't born with your exact drive, Julian. I didn't inherit your energy level, or your impressive focus and commitment that everyone praised your name for at every gym we belonged to. I'm just happy you're finally going to marry your female twin so you'll never have to live with such disappointment and unfulfillment in your life again."

"Whit, I never disregarded the times you tried, but there was a lot of lying often mixed in with all of your trying. I can't even recall all the times we went to doctors and specialists to see if it was hormonal issues, or thyroid issues, or water retention, or some random disorder causing your weight to mysteriously increase," he scrambled in frustration to stack his words as he often did in our disagreements. "Thousands of dollars spent in hundreds of medical visits, only to discover that the main issue of the issues was your stashes of crappy snacks and junk food hidden all over the house. You were hiding everything because you couldn't control your cravings, despite the issues we were already fighting with your soaring blood pressure, frightening bouts of sleep apnea, and chronic fatigue that had you longing for a nap even at the start of the day."

"Lots of lying? Yes, I lied at times. You lied too, Julian!" I shot back. "Let's not pretend your steroid use wasn't as big a deal as my simple snacking—the snacking you gave me the cold shoulder about for weeks as I tried to understand your issues with your steroids. I'm thrilled you're done with all of that now, but I even searched amongst colleagues for answers to alternatives to the trash you were putting in your body. Yet, unless I was chomping down veggies or gulping smoothies all day long, or waiting for you in my workout gear when you got in from the office, I was blacklisted by my superhero husband. You were the superhero who found no use in a wife who could no longer be a vigorous workout buddy, a peppy play bunny, and sexy supermom every damn day."

"Whit, we can go on back and forth for hours about the drama of us, but it's pointless. It's pointless because it's over. It was over way before it was officially over," he replied with more aggravation as his facial expressions pleaded for mercy. "All we can do now is make the best of it. No matter how much you still hate me, or how much you hate your life without me."

"Hate my life without you?" I gasped with full-blown nausea at the narcissism in his statement. "I don't hate my life without you, and I actually don't hate you, Julian. I hate how much time I wasted in our marriage hating myself for not being the perfection you wanted and slightly demanded."

"Argh! Here we go again!" Julian threw his hands up from the counter in a proclamation of surrender. "Whitney, you're not a victim. You weren't a victim when I first met you in college complaining about your weight. You weren't a victim when we both left our marriage that had already been over for years. I hope for Christ's sake this is the last time I'll have every detail smeared in my face again about how I spent some of the toughest years of my life trying my damnedest to be understanding about every issue surrounding your weight even before we met and married. I am not Superman. I'm as human as the human I married and unfortunately divorced," he continued on fervently. "If we're ever going to really get on with life and make sure that the 11-year-old life we created together has a good chance at having a happy and healthy life, we've both got to get our shit together in this constant back and forth schoolyard type fight of who ruined whose life."

"Unfortunately divorced? Wow, you're not as senseless as you've often seemed to be over the past few years," I laughed, attempting to change the tone and direction of what I knew was the ending of our conversation. "Well, as long as you know what you lost in letting Whitty go."

"You are ridiculous, Whit!" Julian laughed heartily at my facetious comment. "You know what I meant, and you know that I mean it. I want all of us to be okay, especially our baby girl."

"I know, and we will be. One choice at a time," I assured. "So, can we begin being okay with officially deciding this wedding trip won't be a full 10 days of distress for Emmy?"

"Yes, I'll agree with that," he smiled and kindly nodded with his response. "Only under the condition you keep at it with your fitness program. That's brought a bigger smile to Emmy's heart than you probably know. I've actually never heard her sang her mom's praises louder than mine."

"Really? Well, I guess our baby girl really is growing up to be just as smart as me," I teased back, swelling with dignity in what the past couple of months had already meant to me personally. "So, how does it feel to be number two now, muscle man?"

"Ha-ha! I wouldn't know. I'm still taller than you are. My skin tone is still a better shade of olive than yours will ever be. And, I'm sure I still have a few less gray hairs than you've had to dye in your mess of long locks," Julian laughed out loud again as I chuckled with a calm that made us both smile even more.

"Omigosh! It's so much fun working out with you now, Whit! I could barely breathe over here. I know my heart rate went to zone 5 at least ten times, though my monitor read differently," Olivia chuckled as we set our stair climbers to cool down mode.

My cardio had improved immensely over the past few months of working out with Cory and his programming. The days of being near death at warmup mode was not only history, but I also actually looked forward to my cardio days. Those days were spent with either Olivia or Barb, depending on whose schedule paralleled with mine, or who I needed to catch up with on the details of life and everything in between. As my weight continued to decrease while my energy and consistency continued to increase, my relationship with both of my best of friends was better than it'd been in quite some time, even though Olivia had always been on my good side when I'd barely had one.

"You did great as always, Olivia! I was also a little surprised at my energy level today. After all the punishment Cory put me through this week, I'm happy to be able to almost walk normally much less push through the intervals in today's fight on these relentless stairs," I laughed in response.

"I'm just so proud of you! I mean... Wow! You're not only looking good chica, but you look good doing it," Olivia laughed with complete admiration for me in her voice and on her face. "Do you remember how many times you barely got through the first ten minutes of our cardio workouts before giving me one of your *damn you to hell* looks? Then, you'd disappear and double dare me to even attempt to ask why you hadn't come back to finish up?" She laughed even more. "How much have you lost so far? It looks like close to 50 pounds!"

"I've lost 52 pounds as of yesterday. I can't believe I weigh under 200 pounds now. For the first time in over a decade, I feel good about what I'm doing in my own skin," I could feel myself smiling from ear to ear while answering her question. "We're a little over a week away from wrapping up my first 90 days of training, and I'm so shocked on so many levels, Olivia. I'm amazed that I've accomplished so much, and then again I can't believe how much time I spent convincing myself I couldn't accomplish anything. The more I brag on Cory for everything he's done to push me and really believe in me, the more he reminds me of what I've really done for myself."

"Whit, I agree with him. You ultimately made the decision to transform your life, and you're doing the work. Just watching who you've become during this process has been amazing," she beamed at me. "I mean, you were practically smiling throughout our entire workout today. And oh my, your nutrition! I thought I was going to die when we were at lunch last week, and you completely passed on the bread basket, twice. Your plate was loaded with every veggie you could get your hands on. And, you drank water only. Water! I don't know where you buried the old Whitney, but you'd better keep her there, chica!" She finished with a roaring laugh.

"Ha-ha! Old Whitney still tries to creep in, often," I laughed, acknowledging the truth of my continued battle with complete honesty. "However, I'm finally realizing it's not worth it to trample all over my progress anymore. The way I feel now is priceless. Not to mention, how I look. It's so worth it to really keep at it. All of my results have come just

113

by eating cleaner and working out like I mean it. I was just thinking this morning after finishing breakfast and dashing out the door with Emily that it's been mostly the changes Cory's challenged me with in my daily nutrition that's been the hugest key to getting such solid results. And, those changes have also helped me sustain the energy I've needed to get through the work of all of our tough workouts. Even when I want to throw all caution to the wind on a cheat day, I can hear Cory's annoying preaching in my head: *'You can't out exercise awful nutrition, Whit. Food is fuel for the body. Feed your body how you want it to function—completely well, or in complete hell,"* I laughed at my attempt to impersonate his deep, smooth voice.

"I have to admit I've stolen a few of the tips you've told me about what he's given you," Olivia giggled in confession to me. "After about two solid weeks of really watching my sugar content, even with my favorite fruits, I lost 3 more inches! Whit, I was so excited I dropped my skirt, which no longer fit, around my ankles and grabbed my phone to call and tell Paul about it immediately. He was annoyed I was actually interrupting a business meeting, but I told him he was either going to smile briefly through the phone about it, or get ready to wear a serious frown when I don't let him touch me in the new dress I'll be flaunting my new waistline in at his company party," she giggled even harder at her facetiousness towards her husband.

"Ha-ha! Steal away my friend! Cory's been so correct about so much. Even his initial strategies of making sure I eat every three hours to eventually speed up my metabolism actually worked. I still can't believe I'm eating all damn day! I go from meal to snack and another meal to another snack. Then again, I've lost far more weight than when I would eat much of nothing all day and later chomp down on everything I could get my hands on at dinner," I laughed out loud at my not so distant memories of the many wake up calls I'd experienced in my fitness journey. "I thought he was seriously trying to make me fatter than I already was, or just incredibly nauseous all day long. I fought him so hard on my meal schedule at first. I fought him on pretty much everything, but his insight has worked miracles on the mess I was making of my body and my health."

"I totally remember, Whit. You called me saying you were thinking about firing him so that you didn't end up setting his entire desk on fire, along with all of the to-do lists he was overloading you with," Olivia laughed out loud as she recalled another moment of my moaning and groaning through the growing pains I'd somehow learned to grow up and endure within my fitness journey.

"Yep! Now, I've found myself telling him I might design a cookbook with the huge treasure chest of information he's helped me with," I replied with a laugh full of conviction. "Who would've thought I'd be eating veggies with literally every meal and eliminating bread and all its cousins at

115

most every mealtime? I'm replacing everything fried with everything broiled and steamed and sautéed. I'm drinking water like a fish, and I'm eating fish as if my cherished rib eye steaks no longer exist. I'm eating sweet potatoes and brown rice in place of my signature mashed potatoes and gravy and creamy fettuccine alfredo. I'm even watching the grams of sugar I eat in everything and choosing not to add salt to anything. I've cut back so drastically on dairy that my once beloved lattes tastes like paste on my pallet," I continued on with the preaching mode I often teased Cory for utilizing. "And Olivia, I take more vitamins and supplements than I do meds now as my blood pressure is back to normal, my glucose readings are in normal mode, and I'm actually sleeping through the entire night."

"Omigosh! Whit, so you mean that..." Olivia exclaimed.

"Yes, I have another doctor's appointment next week to officially confirm where my health profile is, but it's already so evident I've gotten my entire life back!" I interjected, trying my best to withhold my happy tears. "For the first time in my life, I really do see this as a lifestyle. I'm so over the roller-coaster, Olivia. My weight has been more up and down than a kangaroo in mating season. I'm finally realizing it doesn't have to be that way."

"So, you completely get that being fit is an actual lifestyle, and it's not about a quick diet just to flaunt a new style that's almost out of style by the time the exhausting diet is over?" Olivia roared in laughter after repeating her wisecrack statement she'd mentioned to me many times before.

"Yes, I'm finally getting it," I chuckled. "With Cory standing over my face twice a week and stuck in my head 24/7, I'm getting the fact I can't simply rest on my laurels at every stage of progression and success. I still have about 50 pounds to go before my body and health is really where I know it can be. It's not just about the difference on the scale, or in the size I want my clothes to be anymore. Nevertheless, that'll always going to matter to me as long as I breathe woman," I laughed even more while being completely honest with Olivia and myself. "It's also about how I want my joints to feel, as my active years are clearly not over. I want my energy level to be okay even when my hectic schedule has me almost too busy to focus fully. It feels great to finally not be so stressed out and annoyed at everyone around me just because I'm so overwhelmed and disappointed at myself because of what I know I'm not doing to take care of myself," I continued on in complete honesty of my life's details. "It feels fantastic to know Emily has a good example to look to in her mom now. I want my baby girl to know that when I say I love her and I'll always take care of her, she can have complete confidence that I mean it not only because I'm her mom but also because she sees how much I love and take care of myself."

"Aye! Just the conviction in your voice is making me tear up, Whit," Olivia smiled as she quickly brushed away the tears falling through beads of sweat that were still evaporating. "And you're not only going to lose those next 50 pounds, but you'll also be even stronger and more secure than you are now."

"I think so too," I agreed with a confidence that was beginning to feel normal on the inside of me. "I was so afraid at first of Cory challenging me to workout for 30 days solo, with his programming, after our initial 90 days are completed. Now only a week away, I'm in full throttle mode, especially since my crush on him has only grown through every crazy session of everything."

"I told you from Day One that I knew Team Cory and Whitney would eventually be working up more than just a sweat," Olivia laughed in her instigating matchmaker mode.

"Argh! I wish. I just don't know if I'm his type. Even if I were, he's been so professional. Although we've always been playful, he really keeps it under control. So much so, I'm sure he's completely missed everything I'm not even good at hiding," I responded, slightly wondering if Cory ever noticed the few hints of interest I displayed despite my fears of utter rejection. "At least I've stopped twirling my hair so much in between sets of work, trying to make sure my posture is always in perky mode. His workouts keep my shoulders way too sore for those shenanigans anymore," I laughed.

"I've already told you, Whit, shenanigans is not what seals the deal. It's all about you simply being

118

yourself, even in the silliest moments. If Cory is as smart as we both know he is, he's already gotten your every message, Whit. He's just wisely waiting for the best time to fully reciprocate all of it, and even more. Just because I'm a grandma now doesn't mean I can't recognize swag. He's got it," she giggled at me with a wickedly funny expression, emphasizing her good use of a hip word.

"You and your trendy words, Olivia," I burst out into complete laughter. "What am I going to do with you and your efforts to fill your cool quotient?"

"You're going to continue to learn from it just as I'm going to continue to learn so many of my fitness and nutrition tips from you, or at least from what you're learning from him," she smiled and winked at me with full admiration. "I'm so proud of you, my friend."

"Thank you. I'm pretty proud of me too," I smiled back at her.

CHAPTER SEVEN

When Surreal Meets So Real

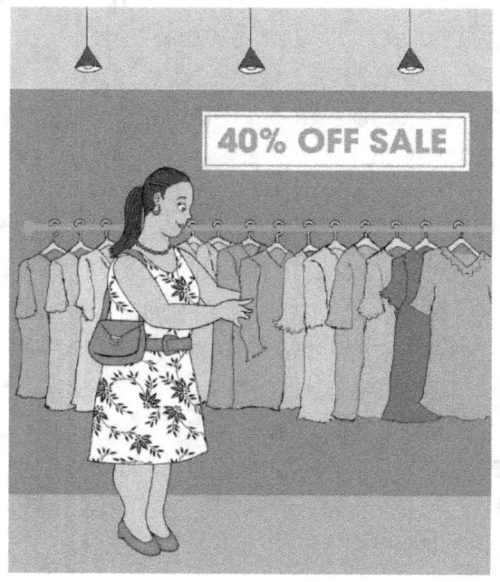

"Thanks so much for coming with me today!" I squealed as Barb and I pulled into a great parking spot in the mall garage.

"You're so welcome! I wouldn't have missed this excitement for anything, Whit. Besides, Rick actually having a Saturday afternoon off to hang out with the boys is complete awesomeness. Then again, I know our nanny is probably doing most of the hanging out and babysitting," she grinned, rolling her eyes in a faux frustration.

"Ha-ha! I'm very afraid of how that game room is going to look when we get back to your house though," I laughed in agreement. "But, let's not even think about it. Nothing's going to ruin this shopping day!"

The fact I was going shopping for smaller sized clothing for the first time in years had me on the brink of tears all morning. More than 50 pounds had come off of my body, and even more weight had come off of my soul over the past few months. I'd become more excited about the whole process than I'd actually been afraid of going through it for years. Every tough session of getting through everything my body still struggled a bit to do was worth it. Every tough moment of saying no to everything my taste buds still tried to convince me to eat was worth it. All of it was worth it to be able to finally shop and live with full energy and full confidence in knowing my weight was no longer the heaviest of burdens in my life.

"Is it all still surreal to you, Whit? I mean you've lost like four sizes, and you're five inches taller in confidence and happiness," Barb grinned with absolute admiration.

"It does feel surreal. If my body wasn't so ridiculously sore every day from Cory's workouts, I'd probably pinch myself repeatedly," I laughed.

"Well, if I haven't already told you a thousand times, I'm so incredibly proud of you, sis. I'm so amazed at you, and I'm so happy for you," Barb beamed even more. "So much about you is so different, Whit! It's hard not to tear up every time we hang out now. I absolutely refuse to though, as you already laugh at me way too much!"

"Ha-ha! I actually wouldn't laugh at you too badly, unless you start the huffing and squealing that usually comes with your deep cries," I teased. "And thank you. You've always been proud of me, Barb. Even when I acted like a big baby in the few baby steps you've watched me take over and again," I admitted with a smile. "If I hadn't already apologized for the thousandth time, I'm sorry for all the hell I caused you as I went through my own personal hell of shame and self-hate. I can't believe how I let my own misery allow me to treat you the way I did for years. Not to mention, how I mistreated myself as if my life and health were of no value."

"Whit, I've already accepted your apology just as you've got to accept it was all a part of the steps in your journey," she smiled. "I knew you'd one day finally get it together and get on board with taking care of your life. You're so strong, and you're so determined when you make your mind up to do something— good or bad," she laughed with her *I know you* look.

"I know," I replied with a silly grin. "And, you know what? I've finally realized that making the decision to make all my exercising and eating well an actual lifestyle has taken so much of the awful struggles out of the overall struggle in it."

"Oh, you don't say!" Barb interjected, teasing me with another bright smile.

"Ha-ha! Really. It's hard as nails to stay consistent at times, Barb, but it feels so damn good to workout because I actually look forward to it, and to eat well because I actually want to do so," I sat up a bit taller in my seat to explain my thoughts further. "Even on the ridiculously hard and exhausting days of trying to continue to do right by myself, I'm able to tough it out because I know the details of my life and my body are worth it," I continued. "Barb, just the way I feel about myself now. I don't... I really don't hate myself anymore. And, I don't hate you, except when you're rocking a pair of heels," I chuckled, refusing to hold back the tears beginning to trickle down my face.

"Ha-ha! Don't hate. Participate," she retorted in complete laughter.

"You and that ridiculous statement! You're cute, but you're so not cool. Leave the cool quotient to me," I giggled at her, patting my tears away with a tissue I'd drawn from my purse.

"Oh, you're so not cool, Whit. You're definitely hilarious at times, but you're not cool. And don't forget, you've got a little over a year to get it together before Emmy becomes a teenager, totally realizing that we're both not cool. But, of course she's always going to kind of think I'm cool because I'm her aunt and not her mom," she laughed even harder before stopping to realize what we were both thinking.

"Wow. Where has the time gone? I still remember crying my eyes out on her first day of pre-school, and now she'll be in junior high soon," I responded with a slight gasp as a new round of tears formed in my eyes. "You know, Cory was just telling me in one of our sessions last week that I can't play the guilt game in my fitness journey because it's a huge de-motivator, but Barb I can't help but think of all the time I've wasted in not being a healthy and active mom for her. Now that she's becoming a young lady, and she's already begun to build a heavy frame, I feel like a helpless hypocrite trying to steer her in the right direction now. Just months ago I fought her bitterly at first on agreeing to do that Fun Run which ended up being one of the best times we've had together since the divorce. I just can't..."

"Oh, no you don't!" Barb interrupted with a fierce charge in her voice. "The only thing you can't do is spend any of your progress reflecting on everything you feel you've done wrong with Emmy. Whit, the only point you need to have your focus on is the fact that she's a great kid who has a great mom who adores her and is doing everything that's best for her now. You can't change anything about yesterday. None of us can. The easiest way to screw up today is to continue to live in guilt and regret about yesterday," she stared right at me, trying to maintain eye contact as I seriously wanted to disappear into my printed sundress. "Now that you know better, you're doing better. That's what matters."

"That's the big deal, Barb. I did know better. I knew from far too many solid sources. I'm not trying to beat up on myself. I'm just finally owning the fact that I let my crazy blend of pride and insecurity stop me from applying so much insight and support to my life for so long," I paused a bit to choke back tears yet again. "Every doctor visit that should've gotten me on track merely pissed me off and made me feel even more disgusted with myself. All the things I watched you do so well and so consistently could've inspired me, but it only infuriated me to the point of losing it inwardly and outwardly. How did you ever put up with me, Barb?" I laughed in embarrassment at yet another memory coming to mind of my formerly insolent behavior to all things healthy.

"Like I've said before, I knew you'd eventually come around, Whit. The more I've learned that we ultimately treat other people, including family, how we mostly feel about ourselves, the more I really just committed to try my best to have a lot of compassion on you. However, I did come close to seriously wanting to choke you during our last drama fest at lunch a few months ago. I mean, let's be clear. It's never been fun being the brunt of your mean jokes and awful comments about my small frame, but I knew just from the awful spirit in which you were expressing those things to me, you had to feel so much worse about yourself. The thought of that often made me feel far worse than the blows of your words," she smiled genuinely, her eyes beginning to glisten with tears. "Whit, you know I've been picked apart most of my life about so much malarkey. *'She's way too thin. She's way too pretty. She's way too happy. She's a bit too dark for the white crowd. She's not black enough for the black crowd.'* When you have to fight most of your life to simply be yourself, you learn to be okay with picking your battles carefully—especially with the ones you love."

"Well, I'm totally okay with admitting you're definitely the best of all of us," I responded in genuine awe of how awesome Barb had always been throughout my many bouts of awfulness. "I know we have to get out of this car and start shopping, but I was just thinking back on the time when I got so frustrated with you last summer because you were actually sticking to your fast food rules with your boys even though we were on vacation. I was so mean to you, Barb. Even so, you were so patient with me. You were understanding even as you tried to get your boys to understand they weren't missing out on eating the junk that Emmy and I ate all week at the beach house," I acknowledged, continuing on. "Although your willpower made me want to choke you, I wanted to choke myself more for chugging down trash meal after trash meal. I was already completely miserable for not enjoying our time on vacation because of the weight I was tugging around on that beach, yet I couldn't stop myself from binge eating while bumbling around in complete bitch mode. If I could turn back time, I'd go back and slap some intelligence into myself to help my Emmy understand why she and her mom would've done better eating with you and the boys."

"Yeah, that was quite a week. I was fighting to decide whether to press on and save my marriage after discovering Rick had cheated on me, yet I had to fight it out with you because of the fight going on inside of you," Barb acknowledged with another forgiving smile. "But, we can't go back to any of that, and you can't live in guilt or shame for what happened back then."

"I know," I responded with a half-smile of shame from yet another memcry of the awful behavior I knew I was ultimately paying for in my plight with Emily. "I'm just so concerned for Emmy now, Barb. One of the hugest wake up calls that caused me to get my crap together with my health and weight was when she blurted out that kids at school were beginning to tease her because of my weight, while already teasing her about hers. It broke my heart to know that my darling, who I'd do anything to protect, was being attacked because of my choices," I confessed with full recollection of the awfulness I'd felt in that moment.

"Wow. I'm so sorry, Whit. You never told me that. When..."

"It was on the same day you finally let me have it at lunch. After everything I'd said to you, while blowing off so much of your help and advice, I surely wasn't going to rush to let you know my kid was being teased on the account of her mom being an out of control chunker," I laughed to keep from tearing up even more.

"Is she okay? Has it gotten worse? What have you...?" Barb rambled on a bit frantically with questions.

"She's okay overall. Emmy's far more tough and popular than I ever was at her age, but kids are far more cruel and vicious now. Most of the cheap shots about my weight and her weight have come from her own little girlfriends who've insisted they're just kidding. It's the only thing they can pick her apart about since she's such a leader with her dad's stature and my cheeky personality. I can just sense how confused she is right now though," I continued trying to explain the millions of concerned thoughts racing in my head. "Barb, all her life she's watched me fight her dad and so many others on most everything concerning healthy and fit. Now that she's completely approaching the stage where she's starting to paying attention to her image, she's kind of wondering 'what the hell'. That's the reason we ended up doing that Fun Run months ago. Emmy's not into running, but she told me she knew if she hadn't signed up, it would've solidified the fat girl status a few of her friends have been trying to brand her with," I continued with as much strength in my voice as I could muster through the sting of knowing Emily's pain. "I know she hasn't hit her growth spurt yet, but she's already at 140 pounds on a 5-foot 1 inch frame. While I know it's not morbidly obese for an 11-year-old, it's a real foundation to build the house of cards she's watched me deal with. I just have to find the most non-hypocritical way to steer her well on how to eat nutritiously and be active for all the right reasons. All she's seen is how I've been up and down and back again. She saw me push away every opportunity and warning to live healthy when I was with her dad. She knows that I helped to ruin our family by being determined to continue my destructive behavior and habits. She also witnessed quite a few of the fights that I'm certainly not proud of."

"Whit, you've got to be just a bit easier on yourself in this, or you're going to make it even harder for the both of you. Emmy loves you, and she trusts you. You and I both know she doesn't see you as a hypocrite. Maybe a bit crazy, but not a hypocrite," Barb attempted to make me laugh a bit in the somberness that had settled over our chit-chat. "Simply stay consistent with her, and with yourself. This is still the beginning of the rest of a really amazing life for you and your amazing kid. She'll be okay, and you'll be okay. You just need to know and decide that first."

"Argh! Do you piss sunshine, Barb?" I laughed teasingly. "I don't think I've ever gotten negative advice from you. Even as a teenager, you'd always remind me to keep smiling because 'People *that smile can get through anything.*'"

"Well, it's true!" She laughed. "However, if we don't ever get out of this car, we won't be able to get through a great day of shopping. Not to mention, we have to find you at least one awesome outfit to rock whenever you and Cory finally decide to start dating."

"Oh, shut it! I can't believe you're still on that. He's my trainer. And, he's a very professional one," I gave her the meanest eyes I could muster up to keep from completely blushing at the thought of such a dream ever coming true.

"Oh, he is professional. He's so professional that he conveniently set up the next 30 days of your training program with him to be done on your own, so that when he decides to make a move, it technically won't be as taboo," Barb giggled as she untwined the plot which had been steadily growing in her head ever since I first told her of my sessions with the very single and very hot trainer she and most everyone at Dynamo Fitness knew and loved.

Cory had been divorced for a few years by a woman who had no patience for his schedule or his passion in his fitness career. Though he'd openly shared with me that he'd mostly been a wreck after the divorce, the fact they hadn't had kids together made the break just a bit easier. Although we'd allowed ourselves to playfully flirt a bit, it was often interrupted by one or both of us doing or saying something a bit more serious or seriously awkward. I sensed, in a hopeful way, that we both knew that each of us was equally terrified of the rejection or even the acceptance of the interest from one another.

"You're pretty lucky I don't hate you anymore, Barb, because right now would be a good time to flick you off!" I teased in response as we walked towards the mall entrance to put the cherry on top of an already pretty good day.

"Oh-oh. Why are we in pouty pants mode today, Princess Whitney?" Cory teased, trying to decipher my abnormally quiet entrance to the workout floor.

"I have a few things on my mind, but I'm okay," I forced a smile his way. "And no, I'm not worried about today being my final day in this phase of training with you. I'm actually a bit excited about using the tools you've shown me to get after it mostly on my own. I was just thinking on my way here of how tired I am of inconsistently winning and losing at this process. For once I want to really succeed at taking care of my health. I want to stay fit for all the right reasons. I'm so exhausted with losing weight yet never quite winning at the process. I've always gained back everything I've lost, only to lose even more hope and confidence in the whole ordeal."

"Oh, so you want a real win?" He smiled a bit awkwardly at me.

"Yes, I want a real win," I retorted with a puzzled look at him, as I wasn't quite sure if he was truly listening or being playfully sarcastic with me. "Seriously, I love that I've gotten such great results over the past few months, but I don't want to do the rollercoaster mode anymore. Cory. I'm done with taking two steps forward and eight steps back as I stomp all over the hard work I've put in by going back to begin a new round of my old habits. I want to know I'm really winning at this process."

"I know you're not kidding, Whit. I see your drive in every session. I can see the results of you keeping that drive going in between our time together," he stared directly at me as we began to toss the medicine ball back and forth to start my warmup. "So, what does a real win look like to you? Be real with me."

"I'm always real with you, maybe too real sometimes," I laughed with a slight blush, recalling a few times I'd endlessly cursed at him in our first few sessions together without wrapping up those rants with a decent apology. "A real win to me means being able to wear clothes that don't look like they were made from a surplus of hotel curtains. It felt great to go shopping with Barb this past weekend and buy outfits I actually like and seriously can't wait to wear because I truly felt awesome in them," I smiled at just the thought of the entire experience again.

"I bet you looked amazing in every outfit," he smiled rather hugely.

"Amazing?" I unintentionally gasped, unsure how to respond to such an incredible compliment.

"Yes, amazing," he affirmed, totally owning his statement with an even wider smile. "Whit, please don't pretend you don't know you're beautiful."

"Well, I know I'm not a troll," I laughed nervously, desperately wanting to hide yet hug him all in the same moment.

"A troll? You're a complete advertisement for your Dermatology career," he laughed out loud, seriously rolling his eyes at me. "Whit, I understand

132

your up and down issues with your weight has mostly made you focus on everything you feel isn't right about you, but you can't disregard something like the fact you're a beautiful lady. You and your gorgeous brown hair with your glistening green eyes. You really are a beauty, with a bit of crazy mixed in. Nonetheless, you're beautiful," he grinned.

"And you just succeeded in seriously flattering and embarrassing me, with a lot of crazy mixed in," I replied with an expression I'm sure was beaming a huge thank you to him despite my verbal response.

"Well, my apologies for making you feel uncomfortable," he responded with the genuineness his smooth voice always emanated. "I'm just keeping it real with you as we talk about your real win."

"You haven't made me uncomfortable at all. I'm just taken back a bit. I haven't heard the word beautiful used to describe me in quite some time. I heard it from a guy who I went on a date with a few months ago. It was hilarious to see how quickly he changed his mind on his declaration as the headshot pictures he saw of me online was nothing like the full package he actually met in person," I smiled in slight embarrassment of making such a colossal confession to him. "It was quite an evening I should tell you about someday."

"Well, it was his loss I'm sure, so you don't have to tell me," he stated matter-of-factly while trying to maintain direct eye contact. "But, you do have to tell me what else does a real win mean to you?"

"Well, a real win is also no longer wanting to hide or even specifically request to be in the back row of a professional or personal group picture because I feel like my size takes up most of the picture," I shockingly admitted such a sore spot in my heart.

"What else?" He prodded on.

"Seriously?" I shot him a playfully foul look, considering my previous statements of transparency were huge ones.

"Yes, seriously. We're just now warming up that brain," he smirked with a *please trust me* look I couldn't resist in his gorgeous green eyes.

"A real win for me would be choosing not to turn directly to food when I'm stressed out or simply bored. I've lost more successes in my fitness journey by stress eating and boredom binges than I can even remember. I just wish my default button had the word ENDURANCE written on it rather than EAT plastered on it," I laughed with full transparency of one of the greatest nemeses in my life's journey.

"I completely understand. That's so many people's struggle, Whit. Men and women alike. The win comes with continued discipline and continually caring enough about yourself to keep the promises you've made to yourself," he responded with full empathy in his voice. "What's another one?"

"That's not enough?" I slightly gasped, trying to maintain my form in our warmup as I started to feel as though I were in one of my toughest counseling sessions with Dr. Lansing.

"It's not about it being 'enough'. It's about getting to the bottom of what really matters, Whit," he continued to toss the medicine ball back and forth to me as he awaited my response.

"Okay," I responded with a little less annoyance, finding more clarity in what he was doing. "A real win for me is going on a great beach vacation and not only taking pictures of my kid, and the amenities at the resort, and the food at every restaurant, and just my toes in the stupid sand—all because I'm far too embarrassed and slightly terrified to see myself in the pictures. It's always been tough enough to look into the mirror at the truth of what I've done to my body by not taking care of it, much less looking at it on a picture. I want that to change."

"Wow, I've never heard it explained like that. That's... that's pretty real," he beamed at my openness. "What else?"

"Seriously? Cory, I ought to..."

"Yes, pouty Princess Whit," he laughed as he interrupted my effort to bail out of the conversation. "We both know there's so much more."

"Well, speaking of pouting. I want to stop pouting each time I get on the scale, and it seems like the numbers aren't changing as immediately as I want them to. A real win for me would be taking that disappointment and shoving it right back into the face of that scale as I know the consistent changes I'm making in my lifestyle will always be far more important than what my overall weight says."

"That's a powerful one, Whit," Cory grinned as he saw the light clearly coming on in my psyche.

"Oh, I'm not quite done with this one, Coach Crazy," I laughed, giving him a playfully rude look for interrupting me. "I want to stop pouting in jealousy and comparison towards other women who seem to be in such great shape and have this fitness stuff under wraps. A real win for me would be finally understanding and embracing the physique and functioning of my own body. I want to be completely powerful in my own skin as I'm totally at peace with what I may think I don't have in comparison to someone else's life."

"That's huge, Whit. And, that's part of the huge difference of you simply losing weight on the scale or also losing the emotional weight holding you back even more than the extra pounds. It blows my mind how much women compare themselves to one another—in rather hateful ways at times too," he shook his head with a stressed smile. "Of course men do it on different levels, but you ladies can be pretty vicious about it. Even in hilarious ways it's so vindictive and brutal."

"What do you mean?" I asked hesitantly, hoping he wouldn't peel me apart like he'd done in one of our first sessions when I'd referred to a woman as a 'skinny bitch' when she pranced pass our workout area to hop on a piece of equipment.

She'd strutted about on her long, chiseled frame with such excitement to be in the building that it irritated me all over again to see what's often celebrated past the stubby physique I felt trapped in.

Though Cory didn't humiliate me personally for calling her that, he did make it clear that it was foul. Although I thought it was a rather funny quip, he established it was no less disrespectful than someone choosing to refer to me as a *fat ass*. It was an uncomfortable eye-opener. It was also the beginning of my knowing Cory was the real deal in making sure I would be healthy and fit inside out as we continued working together.

"For example, I had a female client once say in a session to me, *Dogs like bones, but real men like curves.*'" He responded, rolling his eyes back into his head with a mocking laugh, "I was like damn. What if real men prefer both? I'm a real man that's really more into who a woman is on the inside. The bones or the curves are really just a bonus," he laughed even more. "Anyway. One more. Real win."

"Ha-ha! I've actually said that one before, to my cousin Barb. Of course that was a different version of the curvy me," I giggled at how my flirtatious emphasis of the word curvy garnered a good response as I saw a twinkle in his green eyes which made me laugh even more on the inside. "So, last one? Promise?"

"Answer the question, woman, before I make you walk the entire building with this 50-pound kettlebell we're using for the most of your workout today anyway," he teased, picking up the shiny cast iron weight from amongst a few other pieces of equipment he had set out for what he called my 'Evolution workout'.

The fact Cory was planning to have me specifically workout with the amount of weight equivalent to the progress I'd made so far actually had me much more excited rather than afraid. I'd finally drawn a line in the sand with my fitness goals. Whatever it took to solidify that decision was completely okay with me, even if it meant tugging that enormous weight around for the entire hour.

"The most real of real wins for me would be to totally move on with my life in a completely new body and a new mindset without continuing to relive the guilt of what I know was my part in destroying my marriage," I stated with a confidence I'd never held before.

"That's powerful, Whit, and it's doable, especially as you commit to giving yourself complete credit for every win you attain on the way to all the quote unquote big wins," he replied. "I like that you're finally understanding that your win isn't just in the pounds you lose, or the size you eventually fit into, or the outfits you finally get to wear. Your win is in all of the powerful things that you stated. It's also in each and every workout you show up to and finish like you mean it. It's in every rep you complete during every tough set of work you thought you'd never be able to complete. Your win is also in staying with the process not only until you see every goal and aspiration fulfilled, but also until being healthy and fit is a lifestyle and no longer a question of whether or not it can fit into your lifestyle. Am I preaching too much for you again?" He paused to respond to the blank gaze I'm sure was resonating from my face.

"Nope, I've actually grown to like your preaching. I may even miss it a little during these next 30 days of my solo mode," I chuckled. "Just a little."

"Ha-ha! Yep, you like me. And, you're going to miss me. Thank God we'll at least see each other for a moment each time you do your accountability check-in for your workouts. I wouldn't want you going through too many withdrawal spells from not spending enough quality time in my presence," he laughed wholeheartedly as his green eyes lit up with mischief. "Maybe we'll also have to set up a time for me to cook you something from your meal plan objectives."

"Ha-ha! You're as silly as the day is long. You, cook for me? Cory, your schedule is more outrageous than mine," I playfully, yet nervously responded at the slight thought of where our conversation could be going. "Then again, if your cooking is even as close to being as good as you've bragged about before, I may have to take you up on that."

"Oh, I don't have to brag. You can tell by my swag that my cooking is the bomb dot com," he laughed deeply, tossing a corny wink at me to further confirm his attempt at a cool response was indeed void of all cool quotients. "If you like me as I hope you do, and you're going to miss me like I know you will, then you'll have to take me up on it."

"Of course I like you, Cory. You've given me the tools to completely transform my life," I smiled at him, my heart smiling even more at how much he'd grown to mean so much to me in such a short period of time. "Even with your exhausting preaching and tortuous workouts, like isn't even the best of words to describe it."

"Ha-ha! Well, even with your princess pouting and profuse cussing, like is quite an understatement for me too, Whit," he grinned back at me.

"An understatement. Really?" I responded with another solid smile, taking in the gravity of his statement and everything I suddenly realized he may've been hinting to me during our times together. "Well, if I weren't your client, we could both like the hell out of those likes," I finished with a flirtatious giggle.

"Whit, you're technically not my client anymore after today. Of course you'll be freeloading a lot of my insight, but you're on your own mostly. So, we can do whatever we want with our likes, if we'd like to do so," he grinned facetiously with what I was sure was a twinkle in his green eyes.

"Freeloading? How rude!" I laughed heartily with a surge of hope and excitement flooding my face and most every nerve in my body as it became even clearer where our conversation was undeniably headed. "So, I guess what I've sort of hoped about your liking me has sort of come true. Then again, I don't really seem to be your type."

"Not my type? Whit, I told you earlier that this real man likes real women of all sizes. And, let's be real. You've probably sensed I liked you from the day I met you. However, I knew I'd have to give you time to really like and accept yourself first before you would ever truly accept my liking you," he affirmed with a genuine smile and full on eye contact that made my heart flutter even more. "We really should hangout sometime soon though. I know your schedule is crazy at the med spa right now, but I'm sure we can make it happen. It would be great to really get to know you beyond all your pouting and profuse cussing," he teased.

"It would be great to know you beyond your preaching and causing me to cuss and pout through all your abusive methods of training," I laughed, continuing to flirt without abandon. "And, if you really are the good cook you profess to be, it may eventually land you more than a like."

"Eventually? The glistening in your happy green eyes seems to say differently, Princess Whit," he laughed out loud at the blushing expression on my face. "Let's get focused on the rest of this workout before we're both in a lot of trouble."

"Ha-ha! My thoughts exactly," I agreed, fully kicking into my final session with the hugest smile my heart had felt in years.

CHAPTER EIGHT

There's Just No Point

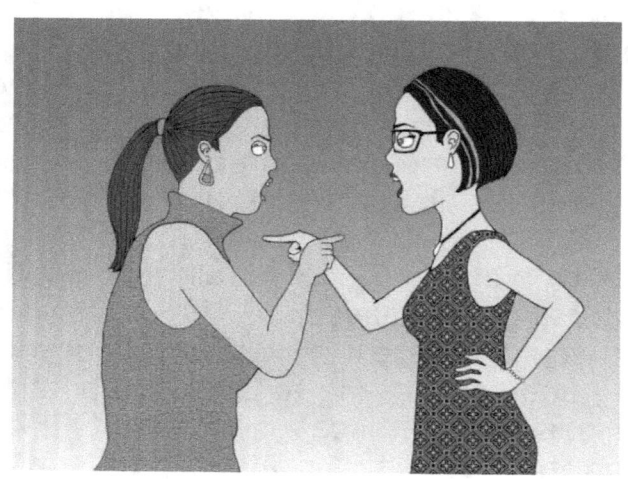

"Mom, can I please go with you when we buy more groceries again?" Emily moaned as she rummaged inside of the pantry.

"You can always shop with me Emmy, but we've already discussed in detail what is and what isn't going to be in the pantry or the fridge anymore," I responded with sheer exhaustion and slight dread of having another pre-teen disagreement of what Emily thought about my new-found commitment on shopping fit and healthy.

I'd a ready rushed home to prepare a decent meal we could both agree upon. After an incredibly exhausting day of multiple laser treatments and multiple meetings about new treatments we'd be implementing at the med spa, I just didn't have the energy to combat the frustrated energy of a snarky kid who just didn't get it and had no interest in finding out how.

"I know we've discussed it, Mom. It just sucks that you're worse than Dad and Miss Karen with all the healthy stuff now. I mean, I'm happy for you and how you've changed, but it's making me miserable. I didn't mind eating all the health food crap at Dad's, but now I have to eat it all the time at home too," she bellowed on. "You don't get hot pockets or corndogs any more. And the fake potato chips you've started buying make me want to hurl."

"Emmy, I'm not ruining your life by bringing healthier food into our home. I totally get why you're so irritated about it. I've spent way too many years having you think that all the junk and fast food we ate was actually okay for us. However, in order for us to both be really okay now, the changes I've made for us are here to stay," I replied with as much patience as I could muster up in my voice. "Let's not forget, I still allow you quite a few snacks, and you have your pizza night every week with every weird topping you want—including your pineapples," I laughed in hopes she'd calm down and realize life was in fact getting much better for her.

"And I'm sorry, Mom that you having a huge crush on your trainer is crushing my life now because everything he says is pretty much the laws of God to you. You eat sandwiches with lettuce instead of bread. You're always double-checking everything in that folder of stuff you've collected from his fitness expert brain," she hissed at me with a huge dose of contempt. "You didn't listen to Dad's advice like that. I totally remember."

"Okay, young lady. I can understand your frustration, but you and I both know you're pushing it now. Do you really think that you being condescending and throwing bad memories in my face about times with Dad is going to help you get your way? In any way?" I responded in full-blown Mom mode. "I know this new lifestyle is all a total shock of non-fun for you, but just because you're in such pain about all of it doesn't mean you have to be a pain, Emmy. The choices I'm making is best for the both of us. I've told you many times over the past few months, you've been my biggest inspiration in all of this. That makes me more determined to continue on far more than the advice of anyone else in my life."

"I know, Mom. But seriously, all of the changing the way we eat, and being at the gym all the time and even being happy about it isn't just about Cory? It's not about you trying to get him to like you because Dad's getting married to Miss Karen?" She stared right at me with far more curiosity rather than defiance. "You used to hate to go to the gym with Aunt Barb, or anyone."

"What? What's gotten into you, Emmy?" I replied in utter shock at the depth of the words that were coming out of her mouth, apparently having settled in her heart.

"Nothing. It's just that I know you like him. I hear how happy you get when he calls. He calls a lot more than he used to," she responded in way too grown up of a tone. "Mom, I just think that your losing weight is not the only thing making you so serious about being all healthy at home. You've lost weight before, and we went right back to normal. You never took it this far."

"I never took it this far?" I replied with an involuntary laugh at the fact that my child had become bolder at 11 years old than I'd learned to become at 37 years of age. "I agree that I never took it this far. That's why we suffered in so many areas, Emmy. You do remember I wanted to disown you just months ago for bugging me to do a mile and a half fun run. Now, I'm actually hoping we can find another one to do together," I laughed, attempting to transform her pouting into at least a partial smile. "I can't change anything about the wrong habits I taught you before. I'm so sorry for that, but all we've got is today. With the wisdom I'm choosing to use now, I'm committed to making every today count for us. Whatever you think you know about Cory, my liking him has mostly happened because I've begun to know how it feels to really like myself."

"You mean you didn't like yourself before, Mom? You've always seemed pretty cool with being who you are, even when you were kind of mean about it," Emily attempted to explain her shock at my statement. "You know, like how you were to Dad, and Aunt Barb, and Grandma."

"Yeah, some adults can learn to pretend pretty well if we feel like we have to. But, no I didn't like myself very much," I admitted to Emily without the shame I knew would've been there just months before in such a conversation. "That's mostly why I gave so many people hell. I didn't like myself for not having the courage to go through the process of doing the work I'm doing now to take care of my health. It's changed a lot inside of me as I've endeavored to get every bit of this excessive weight off my frame."

"I wish I was more like you, Mom. You just decide to do stuff and you do it, even if it makes your only child angry," she finally let out a slight laugh before rubbing the sides of her head to think through her next words as she often did. "I'm just not that strong, not like I think I can be."

"What do you mean, Emmy?" I pressed in even more mentally to hear the heart of what was clearly frustrating her heart. "What's going on? You know you can talk to me."

"I know, but it's just kid stuff," she mumbled back.

"Whatever the kid stuff is, you can talk to me, Emmy. If it's a big deal to you, it's a big deal to me. Talk to me, pretty girl," I nearly pleaded.

"Well, that's one of the things. I know I'm not ugly, but I don't feel like I'm super pretty anymore. I'm the hugest girl in my group of friends, and I'm even bigger than some of the boys now, even the boys I hope might like me one day," she revealed with more gloom in her voice than I'd ever heard from her. "My group of friends aren't as nice to me anymore because I don't really look like them, and I'm not trying to tear myself apart to fix it either."

According to her last pediatric checkup, Emily's 5'1" frame was already carrying 140 pounds, and she had far more fat present than muscle. Her only activity was whatever was required in her gym class or during weekends with her dad, if his schedule allowed. Her doctor warned me she could soon be a candidate for childhood obesity, ultimately leading to juvenile diabetes. Though I'd fought gestational diabetes when I carried her, I'd never made any of it a huge deal to her. I continued to believe that since she was clearly taking on her dad's height, she would continue to grow pass the extra pounds without excess weight being a huge ordeal to her. It seemed my assumption could be wrong as her frame continued to expand while her desire to constitute good health and nutrition decreased, despite the adult voices in her life. Just the thought of watching Emily fight my exact struggle with weight at her age was more unbearable than the scare of having to hear a sure-fire 'I told you so' from Julian or my mom, or both.

"Emmy, I'm so sorry," I affirmed, trying to conceal the frustration already boiling in my blood. "Middle school can be tough because everyone's trying to figure out who they are while trying so hard to be like everyone else at the same time. Sometimes the toughest lessons of this can come from those whom you first knew as friends."

"I know, Mom. It's not just the stuff they say, but it's how they say it," she continued on, trying to appear strong about it. "They used to make comments about your weight, and now that they've seen you've lost quite a bit of weight, it's all turned completely on me. They tell me it looks like I may be drinking a secret potion in my sodas to transfer all the weight that you're losing to my body. They think it's so funny. I mean, Lexie was like a sister to me, and now she's the ringleader of all the jokes."

"Lexie!" I responded without concealing the shock or anger I felt in realizing she was not only Emily's best friend, but Emily had also stood up to rounds of bullying Lexie underwent in their previous school year. "Maybe I should speak to Tracy about it this week. I definitely don't think she'd agree with such behavior from Lexie, especially being that you've stood up for her before in the face of heckling and teasing."

"Mom, I know. But, you know Lexie hates her mom and her dad. She also doesn't really listen to them." Emily reminded me of a truth that had always annoyed me about The Clarks. They'd been such great friends to us that I consistently chose not to judge them. I'd tolerantly decided to view Lexie as just a bit more spoiled as an only child than I'd allowed Emily to be. "If you go to Ms. Tracy about any of this, it'll only make all of it worse."

"Maybe at first, but it could definitely stop her from going way too far, if she already hasn't," I searched Emily's fully strained face for a response.

"It's not always super mean. It's just the way she says some of her stuff. She hisses at me like she's been waiting forever to say it," Emily continued on. "We had pizza and a salad bar for lunch today. Although everyone in our group was grabbing two slices, she looked at me and told me that I would look much better piling my plate with cucumbers instead of getting ready to inhale an entire pizza. She saw that I was only getting one slice because I don't even like our school pizza."

"Wow. That is mean, Emmy," I confirmed, determining whether or not to offer her ammunition to use for what could obviously be a next time. "What did you say to her in response?"

"I just told her to mind her own business about what I put on my plate because at least my food seems to be working for my boobs," she responded matter-of-factly.

"You told her that?" I responded with a sense of pride in my voice, trying my damnedest to hide the smirk I knew was plastered on my face.

"Yeah. I think that's one of the reasons she's started treating me differently. I mean I don't like having to wear a sports bra in gym class already, but I know she hates on me because she doesn't even need one. She probably never will," Emily smiled a bit as a light bulb seem to go off even more on her situation.

"Did she back off after that?" I pressed on for more details.

"Not really. She actually said something to the other girls like, *'Emily's being sensitive today, but she knows I'm just kidding. I know she can take a joke because big girls don't cry. Right, Emily?'* I just replied *'No, they don't cry, but if you don't back off, they'll bite.'* You know, like you used to say to Dad and Aunt Barb." Emily said with a smile that made me know somehow she would still come out on top of the madness whether I decided to intervene or not.

"Yes, I did say that quite a bit. It was mostly to cover up how much I was really hurting though." I admitted to her with a vulnerability I was no longer afraid to hide from her. "Emmy, I'm glad you're standing up for yourself, sweetie, but you don't have to pretend it doesn't hurt you as you deal with their behavior. You can chat with me to get through the sting of it. I've been there. And, what's just as important to know is that what you're experiencing is not how real friends treat each other. Do you think it's maybe time to find a better group of girls to hang out with? You're way too smart and too awesome of a girl to waste your good times at school with anyone who doesn't treat you as amazing as you are, even if they were a good friend to you at first." I stated in a voice I hope conveyed I wasn't just being her mom but also her friend.

"I know, but the kids who are smart like me are also kind of weird, in a not so good way. The kids who are kind of cool and awesome seem to think they're so awesome. I think Lexie is trying to become the leader of that whole group of them anyway. I wish I could just grow up right now and go straight to college in New York, leaving all these juveniles here to window-shop with their moms," she laughed at what she knew was a completely silly grown up thought.

"Well before you head to New York, we have to get some dinner into your system," I laughed with her. "Are you up for some way too healthy stuffed chicken and asparagus? I even have a surprise dessert I know you'll actually like too."

"Whatever you make is fine, Mom. I know you're not trying to kill me with all the healthy food. You're only ruining my life right now with all of it so that I can maybe have a super-hot trainer like me a lot when I'm older," she laughed even more.

"You'll be 30 years old when I even think about allowing that, Emmy!" I laughed as I jokingly shook a spatula at her. "And being that it's been about three weeks now since I've worked directly with Cory, you've got to give your mom credit for sticking to it on her own. I'm down another 12 pounds which is now close to 65 pounds totally lost."

"Mom! That's awesome. I'm so happy for you," she squealed in admiration at me.

"Thank you, pretty girl. I'm happy too." I beamed.

"I'd be even happier if you keep on losing so much weight that Cory will let you start buying hot pockets again when he realizes there's going to be barely any of you left to hug!" She giggled.

"Emmy! You are a mess, kiddo." I laughed out loud. "How did I create such a clone of me?"

"Magic, maybe?" She responded with the adorable smile I'd been waiting all afternoon to see.

"So Mom, are you going to be able to look after Emmy on Saturday or not?" I asked with hesitation as I gave Emily a few minutes to grab the rest of her things in her personal playroom set up at Mom's.

Although I hated asking her to do anything beyond the few random evenings she looked after Emily when my client list extended beyond our normal office hours, I desperately needed her to say yes, as Julian and Karen were going out of town to take part in a couple's weekend to prepare for their upcoming nuptials. Barb and Rick would be out of town to see his parents all weekend, and I dared not ask Tracy being that Lexie was still rapidly becoming Emily's archenemy rather than her unofficial sister.

I couldn't wait to fully accept Cory's request to take me on an official date that weekend. We were finally planning to have a fantastic time beyond our romantic coffee chats and hurried lunches. Over the past weeks, we'd spent much time beyond the gym enjoying more amazing conversations than I could recall having with a solid guy since the early years of my marriage to Julian. Cory was so amazing on so many levels. The details I'd grown to discover about him was more than my heart could contain yet everything it longed for. I was thrilled at how caring and patient he was to allow me the time and space to arrive at a place where I was no longer afraid to fully welcome his pursuit of me. I was also ecstatic about that fact he still encouraged me and only helped me to be tougher when the tough got going in my weight loss goals. It meant so much to know he saw the real me past every pound and every issue I was fervently working on. I was on my own version of cloud nine, realizing more and more that the strength, sass, and confidence which made him like everything about me was what I was also growing to seriously love about myself.

He and I were thrilled to not only be officially celebrating the wrap up of the 30 days I'd been working out solo and lost 16 solid pounds in the entire time frame, but we were also reveling in the fact that I'd be working out solo for good. We both decided that we'd rather our relationship be a mushy version of boy met girl while I continued on with his consistent insight and motivation rather than linger on as trainer transforming his client in complete crush mode. Though we felt like we were way past the age of calling each other boyfriend and girlfriend at 39 and 37 years old, we were excited to officially place a title on what our hearts had been screaming for weeks through every solid chit-chat and soft kiss. Though we were careful not to jump the gun past a few silly jokes, we both sensed our new titles wouldn't matter as much as the one we were obviously heading towards.

"Whit, I told you when you mentioned it to me a week ago that I have an instructor training to do in Houston this weekend. I put off becoming a fitness instructor for years while I struggled and pleaded with your dad to take care of his health," she replied with her typical blank expression towards me. "The whole weekend is already paid for, and I simply can't sacrifice it for the price you're now having to pay in sacrificing your marriage and becoming a single mom. I know you're all excited about this new guy, but if you had done things differently with Julian, we wouldn't be having this conversation that I know you're going to try to make me feel guilty for somehow. I just can't do it this weekend. Next weekend, maybe yes."

"Wow. Mom, I just can't ever win with you, can I?" I replied in full-blown annoyance and shock at the combination of heartless words she'd thrown at me yet again. "Yes, Julian and I are divorced. Yes, I was a huge part of the breakdown of our marriage. And yes, I am moving on with my life as a single mom with a guy who's helped me in more ways than I can even explain. He's inspired me to see who I really am beyond all the weight I've clearly loss. You know, the weight you're still not saying much about," I continued on. "I've dropped almost 70 pounds over the past few months, and you've not only declined to give me a real congratulations but you're also still reminding me of what you think my hugest failures in life have been."

"Whit, I've told you congratulations. I even chatted about your progress with Barb a couple of weeks ago. I told her how pleased I am to see you doing so well in your goals," she retorted. "I'm not sure what else you want from me when we both know that no one's sure how long this exact phase is going to actually last. You've started and quit so many times that I don't know whether to fully celebrate with you, or get ready to cry for you during the next crash and burn."

"Ha-ha! There's just no point," I laughed out loud at her condescending dissertation without trying to hide the tears involuntarily beginning to form in my eyes. "Mom, I don't need you to celebrate with me or cry for me. However, I do have a suggestion," I continued on with more confidence than I'd felt in her presence in years. "During your fitness training this weekend, please try to find out how to truly motivate people who are struggling with this whole weight loss process. No matter who chooses to show up to your classes, everyone won't be as perfectly perfect and fabulously fit as you seem to think you are in your 5'6' frame that carries barely 130 pounds. Fit doesn't happen easily, Mom, nor does it happen in the same way for everyone. So, you may want to become better prepared to deal with those who seem like such failures in your eyes," I continued on heatedly. "Honestly, I'd think that in all of your fitness expertise you'd know that one of the easiest ways to make the mental work of it even tougher is to be around someone who just doesn't seem to get how tough it really is. How can you not realize that the degree of tough is different for everyone, no matter how many times they've crashed and burned or conquered and triumphed?"

"Whit, I didn't mean to hurt your feelings. I was just stating the truth we both know about your experiences. Your dissertation to me about fitness isn't going to make me feel like I've been such a hindrance or problem to you. You've always been the deciding factor of what you will or won't do," she responded with far more resolve than emotion as always. "The fact that Dad's not here anymore to take your side against 'super mean Mom' may be one of the only reasons you're so shocked by my honesty. So, unless you want to talk about anything else, I'm not going to be berated by you anymore."

"Berated? What a term to use by someone who's certainly one of the best at rolling out the worst of it, Mom," I shot back as an internal light bulb came on in a manner that stirred the very fibers of my being. "But, you know what, we have nothing further to discuss actually. In fact, I think I'm going to finally decide to do what Jason was wise enough to do so many moons ago, Mom. I will stay away from the house that haughty built."

"Well, that's your choice Whitney," she responded with barely any response at all. "I'm so done with you blaming me for everything you've experienced. You, and your brother."

"Great. I'm done with you talking at me while making sure that every word you say hurts as deep

157

as the hurt you continuously pretend not to feel about the things you simply couldn't control," I returned through full tears. "Dad was fat. He died from so many issues surrounding that. I've been fat. I'm still fighting to not only change that but to also change how I've felt about myself in all of it so that my daughter will know I truly I love her as I've done a decent job at loving and taking care of myself first," I finished. "And, I'll figure out something with Emmy next week too. Of course if you want to see her, you and I know you're still more than welcomed at Julian's."

"What are you trying to prove by this, Whitney?" She retorted with a slight look of shock. "All of this drama just because my telling you no to looking after Emmy interrupts your plans to date this guy?"

"No, Mom. No drama at all," I responded matter-of-factly. "Cory and I will still date and see each other. However, if I'm to continue my progress and not 'crash and burn' as you declared, I've got to protect the details of my journey from people who simply don't believe in me. Even if those people include my own mom, I have to be courageous enough to do what's best for me."

"You are still so dramatic, Whitney," she shot back. "After all these years, still so dramatic."

"Mom, you haven't seen dramatic. And because I honor you enough to not allow you to see the worst of my truly dramatic behavior, you simply won't be seeing much of me anymore. At least not until I'm able to accept that you simply don't understand that your words mean more to me than your pride means to you," I finished before calling out to Emily to load up the car.

CHAPTER NINE

Little Miss Healthy Pants

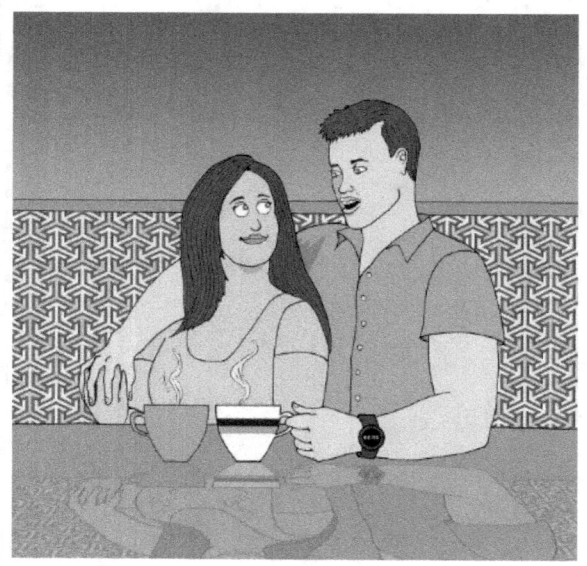

"Are you still planning to join me at lunch, or did you decide to do another lunch of whispering never-ending sweet nothings to Cory again today?" Kristina peeked into my office with a facetious smile to check on me for what felt like the tenth time that morning.

"No, we're actually going to meet up for coffee on Friday morning before he heads out for the weekend. He's just going to use this weekend he took off to spend it with his brother being that they haven't seen one another since the holidays. They're going 4-wheel driving, and they're doing some other silly boy stuff," I smiled at her in response. "He and I are just going to go out next Thursday night since Julian will be picking up Emily a bit earlier for the weekend. Her last day of school and my first day of structured freedom is on Wednesday. Cory's been so understanding and comforting about all the change of plans. He specifically reminded me that we've got too many weekends ahead of us to be heartbroken over just one not working out."

"I like that. As long as you guys are happy, you know that I'm on the happy train alongside you," she smiled back at me as she continued on. "Speaking of happy, have you decided to talk it out with your mom yet?"

"There's no talking it out with her, Kristina. If that were the case, I would've done so when we had our final showdown on Monday evening. Although I don't want Emily to suffer for it in any way, I'm mostly okay with parting ways with her. I've finally realized what my brother totally saw about her years ago. She's a spiteful woman who's only nice to you if you either completely agree with her or if you're so much like her that there's no need to agree upon anything at all," I responded with very little desire to feel much differently about my response. "I've tried my best with my mom for years. I've tried through every putdown she somehow believes is constructive criticism, and every mistake she always feels necessary to smear in my face. Being that I'm now finally at a place in my life where I truly feel great about who I am and who I'm continuing to become, I can't risk losing my sense of confidence in any unhealthy connections, even if that connection is with my own mom. Besides, she's not missing anything in not having me around. She can still see Emily at Julian's. And of course she still has Barb as her unofficial daughter. She's always been good at showing whatever good side she pretends to have to Barb."

"Well, I guess that's the verdict of the jury," Kristina chuckled a bit, attempting to lighten my mood after such a sour diatribe. "Just remember I'm more than willing to help out with Emily if needed."

"I know you are. But remember that I do remember your schedule and life is just as crazy and busy as mine is at times," I laughed. "But, thank you. Just the thought of knowing that someone cares to help is a really huge help at times. I'm just so glad I finally have the energy to get through so many of our grueling days now."

"Right! Do you sometimes wonder how you ever functioned without working out and eating well?" She laughed.

"Oh, no. I don't wonder. It was very clear that I wasn't functioning at all when I was out of shape, especially mentally." I laughed even louder.

"So very true!" She laughed so loud in response it made us both laugh even more. "I'm just so amazed at you, Whit. You don't look or act like anything I can remember just months ago. In fact I think your 'Little Miss Healthy Pants' title is yours to rock now."

"Ha-ha! I'll own it. However, I think I'll just get a new bumper sticker made instead of the tattoo you threatened to get months ago," I laughed in absolute awe of how we'd both become such a better version of ourselves in such a short time. "I'm just so happy about being able to enjoy this upcoming summer in really fun summer clothes and maybe even a real bikini that's not covered in a curtain styled frock for once in my life," I laughed even more. "But you're the one to look at, lady! Aren't you in a size 4 now, or pretty damn close?"

"Yes, closer than close. With the additional 20 pounds I've lost over the past couple of months by tweaking my program with some of the tips you shared with me from the meal plan suggestions of your amazing lover boy trainer, Cory, I'm in the 140's now," she literally squealed at me in response. "Whit, I really can't believe I'm in a size 4! Now my main headache is trying to learn how to shop for such a smaller size. I don't know whether to pretend I can still fit my favorites in the women's section while getting the things I'm accustomed to buying altered, or venture over to the juniors' department. Or, I can go completely couture. I think Rob's credit cards can handle it," she laughed.

"Well, I'm looking forward to having those fit people problems, without the credit card statements," I laughed with a very happy heart for her. "I still have a few more plateaus to cover, but I have to say my shopping trip with Barb weeks ago was one of the best motivators ever to keep me going full throttle. Just the thought that I was in a size 20 only months ago and I'm now able to fit comfortably in a size 12 absolutely blows my mind. I don't know if I'm more excited about the weight I've lost or all the joys I'm finding in losing all the weight."

"Let's just say it's a combination of both," Kristina winked. "And by the way, remember how I told you Rob seems to finally be much happier and proud of how much I've changed? Well, he informed me last night that he's booked a cruise for us in July. I reminded him our anniversary isn't until October, but he said he couldn't wait that long to properly thank me for giving him the gift of having the hottest wife amongst his colleagues."

"Ha-ha! That's more proof that it takes a little more than home cooked meals for a man to function well," I laughed out loud in full admiration of the happiness I knew she felt. "That's so amazing compared to where you've said you guys were just a year ago, Kristina."

"It is. But, can I tell you the ultimate joy in all of it?" She beamed.

"The sex is so much better?" I teased, knowing how prude she could often be in our girlie conversations.

"That too!" She retorted, desperately trying not to blush. "Actually, it's who I've become throughout this entire transformation, Whit. I barely

165

recognize who I am now, yet I know the strength, confidence and wholeness I sense inside of me has always been there just waiting to breathe in full bloom. I think the more Rob saw how confident and happier I was becoming despite the awful decoupling that had been occurring between us for years, the more it sort of gave him a wakeup call. He mostly communicated that to me last night when he saw how stunned I was at his well-planned surprise of such a great trip."

"Wow. I'm so happy for you guys. I still don't understand why I never quite had the motivation to fully do what it took to get my health in order when I was with Julian. I really wanted to try so many times," I reflected out loud. "However, if all my mistakes were made to simply become connected to the amazing man in my life now, that's more than enough reason to just continue enjoying the journey."

"And to enjoy it without any overwhelming regrets of a past that can't be changed," she finished my thoughts with a smile. "So, we'll head out of here at about one o' clock or so?"

"Yes, that's perfect. That should give Mrs. Reardon more than enough time to talk my head off after her facial," I laughed as we exchanged our office version of our *God help me* look.

"I can't believe I'm already thinking about how much I'm going to miss you this weekend," I confessed to Cory as we sat especially close for comfort at our favorite table in our favorite coffee house, Chug's.

Chug's was one of the only places we could escape to for more than an hour without Cory and me running into either of our clients. My clients were always too eager to chit-chat aimlessly when they ran into me in public, sensing they'd hit the jackpot of discovering I had a personal life beyond the med spa. Even so, it wasn't as odd as when we'd run into one of Cory's clients whose blank expression on their faces declared I'd stolen their jackpot opportunity of dating their formerly available hottie of a trainer. Our retreat at Chugs was perfect. We enjoyed each other's company in a simple yet charming atmosphere lined with rustic cabinets filled with real coffee mugs to savor our beverages in the spacious seating areas that were as cozy as our heart to heart chats required.

"I'll be back before you know it, sweetheart. Besides, it'll give you a little more time to let Emily know how excited I am to officially meet her next weekend. That's going to be great," he continued with a real excitement in his voice. "I wish things had worked out differently this weekend too, but everything happens for a reason. We'll just make the best of it until we have the best time mostly all of next week."

"Hmmm. I love how positive you are," I smiled at him.

"I love how positive you inspire me to be," he grinned back with the glistening in his green eyes that always melted me.

"I inspire you?" I teased. "Good to know I'm finally contributing to some part of our relationship, Coach Crazy."

"Ha-ha! Your modesty is not based upon honesty at the moment, sweetheart," he tapped his finger on my nose playfully as he replied. "You know that your encouragement is wind in my sails, babe. Seriously."

"I know. That's exactly how I feel about you too, handsome," I gazed at him with a calm I'm sure said everything he needed to know. "Can you believe how much has happened between us in just a few months? I mean you've went from helping me to completely transform my life to now being such a part of my life that I'm not quite sure how I ever got through any of my craziness in life without you."

"Awe yeah! She likes me! She likes me!" He laughed, coming halfway out of his seat to do a silly celebration dance.

"Omigosh!" I responded in full-blown laughter. "Only you can turn such a heartfelt moment into a complete laughter fest, babe!"

"Yep, and that's one of the many reasons you like me. Like with a capital L," he continued to grin at me. "And yes, I can believe we're where we're at now in our relationship. Whit, I knew from the moment I interrupted your mad dash to that water fountain that you'd be significant to me. I also knew I'd have to wait until you were seriously okay with yourself before you ever took what I could feel about you seriously. You've been worth the wait though."

"That's so sweet, babe," I squealed as I took in his words with a complete smile to my heart, not to mention my face. "It's just that I can barely believe you really liked me even when I was bigger than the both of us put together, and my bad attitude was even bigger than that."

"Whit, I've told you too many times that your weight was never a huge issue to me. The struggles I knew you were dealing with in your health and your mental attitude about yourself was of course a concern. However, I really sensed what you've finally come to know about yourself. You've always been more than strong enough to do what it's taken to get your life back completely." He responded with the same confidence that always calmed my concerns about the details of what he felt concerning us. "Of course I'm even happier now as you've become such a hottie in your office wear and your gym gear. Still, the girl on the inside is who keeps my heart on full throttle mode."

"Omigosh, babe! Just so you know, my like quotient is going up for you more and more. It's going to be pretty tough for me to continue on just saying that I *like* you if you keep on pouring it on thick like this," I chuckled in complete embarrassment of making such a confession.

"Well, why are you continuing to make it tough on yourself?" He replied, pointedly making complete eye contact with me. "Say what you feel. If it's more than like, just say it. Didn't I already tell you I love you last week?"

"Yes, I think you did. I just didn't know how to respond, so I..."

"So, you blurted out a lame joke like, 'you love stuffed crust pizza on your cheat day, Cory," he interjected with a slight laugh. "How rude. Why do I put up with such treatment? All for the sake of you finally accepting my love and adoration and heartfelt passion and..." he teased in a made-up pathetic tone.

"Stop it. I do love you, babe," I giggled at him.

"Say again?" He teased, cupping both his ears while gazing directly at me.

"Cory, I love you. I love everything about you. I love everything about us and our entire journey together so far, Coach Crazy" I laughed a bit to keep from bursting into the full-blown tears threatening to fall under the weight of the words that had consumed my heart for months. "Even when I hate your good advice, I love you. And, I love how you truly love me and believe in me. I really do love you, Cory."

"Yesss! That was overload mode, babe," he pretended to clap as everyone in Chug's seemed to be far quieter than we were. "I like that. I love that. I can just leave my truck here in Dallas for the weekend and skip all the way to Houston to see my brother on all of those good words."

"Ha-ha! You are so stinkin'..."

"Awesome? Handsome? Amazing? Hot?" He interrupted with another grin. "Go ahead and pour it on even thicker, babe."

"Yes, all of that too," I roared even more with laughter. "What am I going to do with you?"

"Now or later? I don't think the restrooms in here are always pristine, or private for that matter," he smirked as he teased with complete inappropriateness. "Besides, I want that to be incredibly special, so later is definitely better."

"Yes, that's exactly what I was talking about," I giggled, rolling my eyes sarcastically through my continued chuckles. "You are such a man!"

"I'm just trying to take care of my princess, and keep you on your toes at the same time," he chuckled as he continued on. "And speaking of taking care of you, did you get the new adjustments to your meal plan I sent to you on Wednesday? You usually reply right back, so I was just making sure."

"Oh, yes I did. I was at lunch with Kristina when your emai popped up on my phone, and I forgot to respond. Speaking of Kristina, she reminded me earlier that day at the office of how much she's hugely benefitted from all the tips I shared with her which came directly from you," I continued on. "Babe, I still really think you should consider doing something with all your good insight. Kristina's lost about 20 more pounds over the last couple of months after already losing weight in different phases of other programs she's done. Even more, Olivia's done so well with what I've shared with her that she's constantly pestering me for any new stuff she thinks you may be telling me. I feel like I've actually trained them both through you," I smiled in admiration of the man I'd grown to love.

"Ha-ha! That is pretty cool, babe. But, like I've said to you before, it's not really brand new information per se. It's a lot of ro brainers to so many people who already take getting fit seriously. Besides officially getting my nutrition certification completed years ago, I've just taken a lot of time to actually investigate and learn as much as I can from what's already out there and ultimately understand how to implement it into my own training programs," he explained.

"Babe, you act like it's no big deal that your insight's been such a big help to so many people," I retorted, wondering why he often downplayed my kudos of his undeniable impact.

"It's not that I don't see the solid results of my guidance, Whit," he replied. "It's just that I know the information I share is accumulated from so much insight already out there. Vegetables are vital at every meal. Water is as important as breathing. Bread is as unnecessary as the processed spreads we can't wait to smear all over it. It's all just simple stuff that seems so difficult to implement at first. Food is simply fuel for our bodies. It's that simple. So much of it seems so difficult because all we've learned far too well is how to chomp down on anything and everything we absolutely love to eat, yet our body hates to digest. Oppositely, we hardly succeed at forcing ourselves to barely tolerate the meals we can't stand, but our body craves. We just have to realize that we can't fuel our cars far better than we fuel our own bodies. Nutrition affects the functioning of every cell in our body, even more significantly than efficient fuel operates our vehicles."

"Babe, that's what I'm talking about. All your insight is probably a no brainer to trainers and other fitness minded people, but need I remind you that we everyday people have heard so much truth and garbage that claims to be truth that we can often barely discern or remember all we've heard," I persisted on. "The way you explain this seemingly difficult stuff is amazing. Why are you so hesitant to possibly share it with more people?"

"I just don't know if it's as big a deal as you're making it, babe," he chuckled apprehensively. "I agree it all helped you, but you were motivated enough to find out some of that info on your own. You've read other materials, so I don't know that it was just my doctrine, or only my way of coaching you that transformed you."

"Babe, are you kidding me? Don't you remember how confused I was on what metabolism really means. And, I didn't even realize how important fresh and frozen vegetables are versus canned vegetables due to all the sodium and awful preservatives in the packaging. Even the fact that the amount of water we need to drink isn't simply eight glasses fits all baffled me. It completely changed my energy level, and it helped me to get rid of my stress headaches when I began drinking the ounces of water best for my own personal profile. I seriously don't know why you're being so nonchalant about all of this," I finished with what I was sure was flames in my green eyes.

"Wow. You're really serious about this, aren't you?" He laughed with a slight nervousness I'd never quite seen in him.

"Yes, your insight has transformed my life, Cory. It's given me a new outlook on what eating well while we're moving well actually means for our body," I carried on with excitement. "I mean if you don't want to go for it, I'll just do it for you. I'll even do it in your honor if you behave well," I laughed facetiously. "Yep! Maybe I'll name it 'The Little Miss Healthy Pants Roadmap to Robust Health and Fitness'. If it does well, I'll be taking full credit and of course receiving great backrubs from you for the rest of my life, after I return home from every eye opening speaking engagement of course."

"Ha-ha! Little Miss Healthy Pants? Isn't that the name you used to call Barb and anyone else who dared to get on your nerves with excitement about fitness related stuff?" He continued to laugh with a face of astonishment and admiration. "What's happened to you, Princess Whit?"

"Well, I guess fit happens." I laughed as I repeated the same quip that had made me question the sanity of the individual who said it when I came across it in a fitness magazine only months before. "But, I've got to ask you, what's happened to you that I'm practically pleading with you to own up to the value of what you obviously give to your clients? Sure you share material you've studied from others coupled with insight you've discovered on your own. Yet, it's shared in your own skilled voice, and your voice is significant enough to be heard beyond your day to day schedule. What's with you, babe?"

"Nothing... everything," he mumbled in response to me. "Babe, I get that you realize how insightful and skilled I am at what I love to do, but the last time I placed my full life and energy into taking who I am and what I know to the next level, my high hopes were deflated. They were completely deflated by the woman who I'd chosen to be at my side because I thought she'd be at my side no matter what," he continued on with a perplexing defeat in his voice. "As soon as my schedule went into overdrive as media outlets and other significant parties opened doors of opportunity to me, my ex-wife walked completely out the door on me. She said she didn't sign up to be the sidekick of a superstar while watching night fall on all of her own aspirations. She seriously didn't get that we were a team, and my winning in life also meant a huge win for her and vice versa. I just don't know that I could suffer that kind of disappointment again, at least not on that level."

"Wow! Babe, I had no idea," I responded with as much pain in my heart as I felt from the expression on his face and in his voice. "Is that why you mostly shutdown when I press on about how much you could be doing about how amazing you are? I'll back off a bit knowing this now," I assured him with what I hoped was a soothing smile.

"No, it's okay. You haven't done anything wrong, sweetheart. And you definitely don't have to back off," he smiled, assuring me that I hadn't caused him any grief. "You're actually completely on target, and your prodding and encouragement is waking up things in me I should've never allowed to grow dormant. I'm a smart guy though, so I'll get this party started again somehow."

"You sure will, babe. And, I'll be right by your side cheering on every bit of your superstardom," I giggled.

"If you don't stop getting me excited about all things tomorrow, I'm going to be forced to pull you even closer and give you a serious thank you kiss with a promise. You know very well how I respond to show I'm extremely grateful," he grinned with a boyish giggle.

"Yes, I do remember. Just a little bit more excited than your boy, Rocky." I laughed as I reflected back on the time I'd briefly met his 3-year old English bulldog, Rocky. He melted my heart as he'd pounced all over me with puppy kisses. Cory said his excitement in meeting me was totally out of character for him, but even a puppy knows the effect of a kick ass woman.

"Yep! He made it pretty clear he's just as thrilled about you as I am. Of course I met you first, and I do like you more. And, I do have better control of my licking," he flirted on mischievously.

"I would hope so!" I laughed. "Speaking of Rocky, is Sabrina still going to look after him for you this weekend?"

Cory and Sabrina were not only neighbors in their condo community but they'd also become siblings as they'd trained for over five years together at Dynamo Fitness. Cory's decision to have taken her under his wing when she was part of his staff had attributed to her growth as a trainer and the courage to eventually step out and open her own fitness studio over a year ago. She wasn't modest in declaring her continued success was largely in part to his mentoring and encouragement.

When Sabrina had met up with us during a coffee date weeks before, it was clear that although she was a tiny framed woman, she was huge in energy and life itself. Her thin yet toned frame paraded a head full of beautifully and meticulously braided hair and a mouth filled with dazzling white teeth that made her ebony skin even more radiant. Her open heart and warm personality shined brightly through her contagious smile as she congratulated me on all Cory had informed her about my nearly 70 pounds lost.

The passion and positivity Sabrina exuded for her career as a trainer was evident as she explained to me that she was put on earth to kick ass and save names. Those were her exact words. She knew it was her life's mission to help individuals understand that fit and healthy is a way of life. Her infectious sense of humor had us laughing out loud at our table as she shared with us about a training session which had left her and a client laughing out loud that morning. She also had us roaring about the months it had taken for she and Cory to explain to so many who worked with them at Dynamo that it was possible for heterosexual male and female adults to be good friends without expecting or exchanging romantic or sexual activity. Cory's decision to remain close to her and her new boyfriend, Kyle, seemed a wise one indeed.

"Yeah, she's awesome," he replied. "She insisted that it really wouldn't be a bother for her, as Kyle is out of town on business this weekend anyway. In fact, I should get going in a bit. I promised to meet her at her studio space early to drop off Rocky and take a look at a piece of equipment she's looking to probably return to the sporting goods warehouse. If it's not easy to use for Sabrina's hyperactive brain, she's ready to toss it," he laughed.

"Ok, babe. I should actually get back to the spa too. I've got just a couple of more people to see before I wrap up my day and pick up Emily later," I replied with a warm smile yet the same nagging feeling of already missing him.

"Cool. Let me escort you to your vehicle so I can give you the type of goodbye kiss that no one needs to see in here with their cup of coffee, unless it's a piping hot cup," he smirked, knowing I would laugh yet again.

"Let's go, Coach Crazy," I giggled as I grabbed his hand that was already extended towards mine. "Can't wait for this kiss. And the next one. And the next one." I teased with overflowing tenderness in my heart.

CHAPTER TEN

Fit Happens

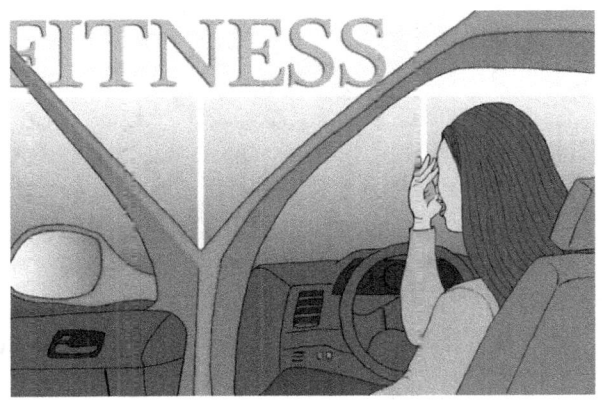

"I know you're not totally excited about going to Dad's for the rest of the weekend, but if I can deal with his last minute change of plans I know that you can find a way to do so too, Emmy," I responded while trying to keep my own temper cool despite the fact my entire weekend had been rearranged as Julian and Karen had not only suddenly announced their change of plans to forego their couples' retreat weekend the night before, but he'd also practically insisted Emily be with him being that it was still his appointed time with her on the weekend. Yet, as annoyed as I felt, I had no plans to ruin a great Saturday morning as I actually looked forward to getting in a good workout at the gym and later doing some solo shopping to get ready for my date night the following week with Cory. I couldn't wait to chat with him later that afternoon to see how his visit was going with his brother being that I hadn't received a good night text from him the night before or a response to mine.

"It's not that I'm not excited to see Dad. It's just that it's so early. Awesome parents don't make their kids get up before 8 o' clock on a Saturday morning. Cory isn't even here this weekend, so why do you even need to go to the gym so early, Mom?" She moaned with a smirk.

"I know Cory isn't at the gym this weekend," I laughed in slight shock of her growing sarcasm. "And, you know that I don't go to workout at Dynamo just to see Cory. We've already discussed that Little Miss Nosy Pants. I like getting to the gym pretty early on a Saturday so I can get on with the rest of my day. Besides, awesome parents don't sit around the house all day on Saturdays, or let their kids do the same. At least not always," I winked at her as she and I both knew we'd spent quite a few lazy Saturdays and Sundays at home before.

"I know," she laughed. "It's just that it's been forever since I've spent a Saturday with you because I'm always at Dad's on the weekends when school is in. I was actually looking forward to spending this whole weekend with you, but then again Dad may not have as much crappy health food at home since he and Miss Karen were going out of town before.

So, hopefully we'll eat out all weekend, at only fried food places," she laughed again.

"I'm sure that Dad and Karen won't be taking you to any fried food restaurants, especially as happy as he's been that you're eating so much better over here now," I laughed out loud at her pre-teen thought process. "Speaking of Dad, he should be here any minute. Go upstairs and grab your bag so that you'll be ready to go when he gets here."

"Oops! I'll have to get my bag in a few seconds because that's him at the door," she squealed with a huge smile as the ring of the doorbell interrupted our chit-chat. "I'll go answer it!"

I didn't dare interrupt her bolt to the door or her excitement. I had no overwhelming desire to be the first to greet Julian's face on what felt like a super Saturday morning with a great day ahead for me personally. Life was finally beginning to feel like I had some confidence and strength in the journey of it all, and I had become rather keen at protecting my new-found positive energy in every facet of it. I not only couldn't believe how much more I smiled for no reason at all but also how much I complimented others for any reason I could find. I genuinely felt happy for most every happy scenario around me.

"Hi, Whit! You're looking great!" Julian interrupted my random thoughts, entering the kitchen will a beaming smile while Emily bounded up the stairs to grab her weekend bag.

"Hi, Julian. Thank you. I'm actually on my way to the gym in just a bit," I smiled back at him.

"Good for you. It becomes an addiction once you start taking it seriously, doesn't it?" He grinned at me, waiting for an answer to match his apparent excitement for me.

"Well, I guess that's a cool way to explain it although I don't know that I'm addicted to it," I smiled oddly at such an odd statement from him especially as we were both aware of the steroids addiction he had fought and won during some of the toughest of times in our tough marriage. "I just see it as a part of my lifestyle now. It's really become a huge part of who I am overall."

"I'm sure this lifestyle has become even better for you to enjoy now that you're dating your trainer, right?" He laughed with more curiosity in his voice than humor.

"I see that our precocious little beauty has been chatting about her mom to her dad," I laughed back at him with no reservation to be nervous or hesitant to answer any of the questions I knew he was dying to ask. "Is there something you're wanting to ask me directly, Julian?"

"Nothing huge really. I was just wondering if you really are dating this guy. And, if you plan on bringing him around Emmy," he responded with an obvious air of disappointment in his voice.

"Yes, I really am dating this guy. And yes, he's actually planning to officially meet Emmy next weekend," I smiled at just the thought of what was ahead for us. "In fact, I was going to make sure it was okay with you that she's with me by Sunday morning next weekend as we both want to spend that entire day with her. I didn't think it would be a big deal for you being that you'll have her the rest of next week when she's released from school on Wednesday."

"Oh, so I guess you and he really are a big deal," he half-smiled at me, searching for more clues. "Yeah, that's totally fine with me, as long as Emmy is totally fine with it."

"Julian, I wouldn't have Emmy meet him if I had any doubt she'd enjoy being around him. Then again, she is your precarious kid," I teased him a bit to lighten up what had quickly become a somber mood in our chit-chat. "He's been a really great guy to me. Although he's been a big deal in helping me transform my life, he's far more important to me beyond that."

"Well, I'm glad Emmy has your smart mouth, so if she does sense something she doesn't like she'll address it pretty quickly," he laughed heartily in his troublemaker mode. "But seriously, I'm glad you've found happiness, Whit. You deserve it. You're a great mom, and you're definitely setting the bar high on life transformations. I mean, look at you. You're disappearing before our eyes, in a really positive way. Being that this new guy is a part of all of it really does say a lot about him too."

"Thanks, Julian. That means a lot to hear from you," I responded with a smile from ear to ear.

"It's a well-deserved compliment," he smiled back at me with an odd look of eagerness. "Are you ready to roll kiddo?" He looked over to greet Emily as she stood at the bottom of the stairs with a smile as huge as her weekend bag. She always packed way too much to go to her dad's.

"Yep! Let me just hug Mom so she doesn't cry too hard when I leave," she laughed as she ran over to me with flailing and open arms.

"What am I going to do with you, crazy kid?" I laughed as I glimpsed at the pleased look on Julian's face as he enjoyed our bond.

"You're going to hug me, and miss me, and count down the hours until you get to see me again," she giggled.

"Yes, that's what I'll do." I teared up just a bit on the inside, realizing once again that life really didn't have to be perfect in order to be just perfect for us.

"Hey, Sabrina. Good morning!" I smiled as I answered my Bluetooth while pulling into my favorite spot at the gym. Although I had no idea why she was calling me rather early on a Saturday morning, the fact that she was a good friend of Cory made her a total friend to me, which is why we'd exchanged numbers almost immediately upon meeting weeks before.

"Did I wake you? I know... I know it's fairly early," she stammered a bit in her voice.

"No, it's okay. I'm actually just pulling up to the gym to get my workout in before I head out to a pretty full Saturday of shopping and overdue solo time," I replied as I tried to bring the excitement level in my voice down to the serious tone I sensed in hers.

"Okay. Well, I apologize for interrupting your day, but I'm really glad I was able to reach you before you head into Dynamo," she continued on with far more urgency in her voice. "I just needed to share something important with you. It's about Cory."

"About Cory? Oh God, did they try to fire him or something?" I responded frantically as I considered whether I should sit tight in my car and listen to her completely before heading into the gym to investigate further. "He had full coverage to take off this weekend, and the parking lot doesn't even seem completely full for a Saturday morning. I'm hoping this new manager isn't nitpicking him about anything."

"No, that's not it at all. But, it is important, and I'd rather not share everything with you over the phone. Can we meet somewhere to chat for a bit?" She continued on with even more anxiousness reverberating through her increasingly faint voice.

"Well, I guess. I'd rather you just tell me what's going on now so I can head in and workout afterwards. Is it so top secret that we can't just chat on the phone about it?" I responded with a bit of annoyance to her secretive and solemn tone.

"It's just that I think it would probably be more appropriate to talk to you in person rather than over the phone about it," she replied as I could sense her trying to maintain her cool without causing me to blow mine as I struggled to quickly uncover the suspense in her words. "I do understand your main thoughts right now are mostly about enjoying your Saturday. So, please know I wouldn't interrupt your weekend if it weren't incredibly important, Whitney."

"Yes, I know. Go ahead, you can tell me over the phone. Important stuff is important stuff whether it's over the phone or in person. And by the sound of your voice, I don't think I'd want to wait another twenty minutes or so to meet up with you and then hear what you have to say. Even if it's because you're probably calling to let me know that Cory wants to break off everything with me, but he's sent you with the perfect words to convey it to me," I let out a forced laugh as I considered the graveness in her voice could very well be that, realizing once again how ridiculously perfect Cory and I's relationship had been from our first official moment of making it official that we liked each other.

"It's nothing like that Whitney, because Cory was never like that," she responded with even more somberness in her tone. "There's been an accident. Cory was in an accident yesterday evening."

"An accident!" I gasped as if I'd been kicked directly in the stomach without warning or relief. "Is he okay? Is... is everything okay?"

"Everything will be okay. But, no. No, he isn't okay, Whitney," she stammered as she virtually whispered, continuing on in her response to me. "Cory passed away early this morning."

"He passed away? What? What... what are you saying? He's... he's dead? Dead!" I began to wail uncontrollably as I tried my damnedest to continue

190

talking to her. "Sabrina, tell me... tell me this is a silly joke... a stupid dare... to get... to get a reaction out of me. Tell me that this crap isn't true. This can't be... this isn't true. This can't be true as I sit here... staring at the building that... that he and I... we built... we built our relationship here," I wailed even more as my broken thoughts and words failed to stop the floods of tears. "Tell me this is a crazy fluke, or some outrageous... mistake in communication. What happened? What the hell... what happened!"

"It's not a joke, Whitney. Not... not at all. I'm still in complete shock too," she whimpered, her broken voice doing little to hide the tears that began to pour from her soul. "His brother called earlier this morning to inform me. He not only knows that Cory and I have been friends for years, but he also knows I've been looking after Rocky this weekend. He even asked me to call George, the Department Head at Dynamo. The family is already overwhelmed by so many calls and details to line out today. That's why I wanted to reach out to you early so you wouldn't hear the news in an even worse manner."

"Oh my God. How... How is this even real? What happened? How did... How did anything happen to him?" I sobbed even more at the thought of how many people's hearts would shatter upon hearing the devastating news. "And his poor dog! Oh, God. Rocky!"

"I know, Whitney. Those were practically the same words I sobbed when his brother called," Sabrina added, trying to keep her composure through her own pain. "Cullen said the state highway report stated that Cory was hit by a vehicle which lost control when he was pulled over to fix a flat tire that happened on his truck. It actually happened just north of Houston. He had just called Cullen as he was finishing up to let him know he'd be running late because of it. He wanted to get the spare tire changed to the signature full sized immediately when he got into the city. You know how much he loved his truck," she explained on. "Cullen is pretty broken up about it too. Even so, he and the family are incredibly thankful the accident didn't happen when they were on the phone. The highway report seems to show it occurred only a few moments later," she began to sob again.

"Oh God! Did he... did he die... right there? On the side... of the road, Sabrina? On the side of the road!" I cried even deeper as my heart sank below the earth that felt as if it were no longer holding me anymore."

"No, he didn't. Cullen said they life-flighted him to a medical center in North Houston but they couldn't... they couldn't stop the internal bleeding," she began to sob even more as she fought to explain. "He said he probably didn't suffer though. They were told he was unconscious the entire time although the medics and everyone involved tried to bring him back to recovery. They tried... they tried everything. The internal bleeding was just too much. It was too much. He had quite a few broken ribs that... severely ruptured his organs as he... took full impact from the hit," she continued with more strength than I could've ever imagined in being a messenger of such news. "And just so you know, the guy who hit him wasn't drunk. It was a completely ridiculous freak accident. He had actually grabbed for something on his passenger side and lost control of his wheel before ne... before he hit Cory."

"How... how could this happen? I just can't... I can't... I can't believe this. God, I loved him. Really... loved him." I pleaded for clarity as I sobbed and screamed from my innermost, having no concern of who could possibly walk pass the spectacle I was most likely making of myself inside of my red luxury vehicle which had become a chamber of total pain yet complete comfort. "What am I going to do? How do I even... how in the hell... how do I deal... with this?"

"Whit, you're asking some of the same questions I've racked my brain w th over the last hour or so. It absolutely sucks. I just don't..." She sniffled as she tried to search for words she and I both knew would never be just right for such a wrong situation. "I know the pain is so much deeper for you, knowing how much you and Cory cared about each other. He was so over the moon about you. He talked about next weekend's plans with you more than the plans he had with his brother this weekend before he left my studio on Friday."

"I can't... I can't even hear that right now, Sabrina," I continued to sob more deeply than I had on the day Mom had called me with the news that we'd lost Dad. "As much as I loved him, and I still love him, that's actually making my heart feel like.... like the same stupid car that hit him... smashed directly into me too. Head first and heart last to finish me. I not only have no freaking idea how I'm going to deal... really deal with this... this awful news, but I also don't even know where to begin... in explaining this to Emily," I cried even harder and deeper as my body shook under the pressure of the grief and pain my heart already felt. "Everything... every breath has been knocked completely out of me. Every bit of happiness I've felt for months has been pissed on... by every detail of this awful news." I bellowed on, feeling as if a damp blanket had been wrapped around my heart and lungs and set on fire just enough to create a thick smoke to gag upon, yet not quite enough to send me into the comatose state I would've much rather been in during such a heartbreaking moment.

"I'm so sorry, Whit. I can't begin to understand how you really feel. I know I'd be devastated if I lost Kyle. Just please know I'm here for you. I really am," she sniffled even more as I felt the sincerity in her voice. "Cory was seriously an only brother to me, and knowing how he felt about you truly makes you my sister."

"Thank you, Sabrina. That means... more than you know," I replied, trying my best to regain my composure and some sort of strength in my voice. "I don't even know how I really feel right now. I feel everything. I feel nothing. I'm just really glad we're talking about this over the phone because I have no doubt I would've collapsed in public."

"Oh, I totally get it. I'd just gotten to the studio this morning to prepare for the day when

Cullen called me with the news. I laid here on my studio floor crying in a fetal position for what felt like more than an hour after I heard it," she replied matter-of-factly.

"Well, carve out a spot for me in there because I'm sure there's still a lot more tears trapped in this broken heart. Hell, get the entire building ready for my blubber fest part two, and three, and twelve," I sniffled a bit more as I made her and myself chuckle a bit. "I just hope he knew how much he was loved. I really hope he knew that."

"Of course he knew that, Whit. That's all he talked about before he left," she confirmed in a voice more kind than I had ever heard from my own mom. "In fact, I keep having to fight the thoughts in my grieving brain that maybe if I had made him leave even earlier yesterday instead of enjoying his rambling about everything he was happy about while helping me, he would've missed being at the wrong spot for the right idiot to hurt him," she began to cry again.

"Oh God! You can't overthink stuff like this, Sabrina. You'll end up even crazier than I am. I'm already sitting here in my car trying to decide whether I want to get out and scream bloody murder in the parking lot or just peel out of here into complete oblivion. Even more, there's a huge part of me that really wants to go inside and retrace all the steps Cory and I always made in Dynamo, kick every piece of furniture and equipment, and then drive off and vow to never come back here again. All because

I can't imagine this place, our place, without him," I began to weep yet again.

"Well, I have a better idea. You don't need to go through the next few hours or so alone in this, especially as you figure out how to inform everyone who knows how important Cory was to you. I can meet you there at Dynamo if you insist, or we can meet somewhere else," Sabrina offered with almost a pleading in her voice. "I've cleared my schedule for the rest of today. I can also fill you in on the details of the funeral arrangements set for Monday morning in case you'd like to be there. I'm sure his dad and brother would love to meet you."

"That actually sounds good. We can either try to find a coffee shop he and I actually never went to together, or I can simply head to your studio. I'd just rather not have any more of my impending emotional breakdowns in public just yet, especially as I have no doubt there's hundreds to come," I replied as rays of hope and helplessness flooded my exhausted mind. "I'll meet you at your studio in about twenty minutes if that's okay?"

"I'll be here," Sabrina responded with what sounded like the sweetest smile in her voice.

CHAPTER ELEVEN

Love, Sweat and Tears

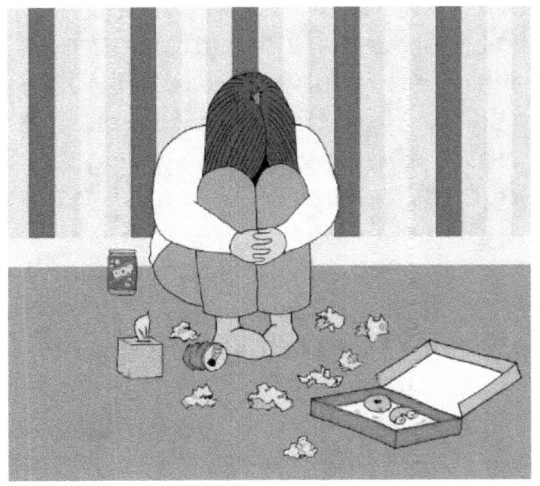

"So, how did the funeral go overall?" Barb asked as her expressions of worry and d sbelief reminded me of the shockwaves continually stabbing through my soul.

"It was awful, and it was awesome. It was awful that it was actually so awesome. There were so many people there, Barb. And the fact that his brother, Cullen, made sure everyone knew me as Cory's girlfriend was so sweet, sc bittersweet." I responded with as much energy as I could muster up after having spent the past day putting on smiles as

I attempted to hold back tears and pouring out tears as I tried to push through to the next smile. "Cory lived his entire life in Houston until his divorce a few years ago. I don't remember even half of the people I met. Sabrina was amazing at putting so many faces with the names she'd remembered from Cory's years of telling so many stories and showing her loads of pictures. Even his ex-wife was there."

"Oh, wow. Was it weird meeting her, especially under those circumstances?" Barb leaned in for a response full of girly gossip.

"No, not really. She's been remarried for over a year now, so it was obvious she was there simply out of respect for his family. No one was neither surprised nor excited she showed. The fact that his mom, who never really liked her for so many reasons Cory said he later discovered for himself, passed away about a year ago probably made it much easier for her to attend," I responded matter-of-factly.

"So overall, it was good despite the clearly not so good circumstances?" Barb confirmed with a question.

"Yes. The speeches and stories went on forever, but it was absolutely amazing to see how many people cared about him and admired him. So many people adored him, just as I did. Clients who hadn't seen him in years were there. Childhood and college friends who knew him way before any of the admirers and recipients of his passion met him were there. They were all heartbroken yet humbly inspired to make the impact he obviously made," I recalled the details as a fresh round of tears began to well up in my eyes again.

"I'm not surprised by any of that. He was amazing. Look at the life he brought back to your life." Barb beamed at me through the bereavement she revealed.

"Please don't remind me," I responded with a half-smile as her words caused my heart to break just a bit more. "You know, his brother told me Cory had felt like I was the one who changed his life so hugely. Cullen said he had mentioned who I was to him before we had officially began training. After he and I had started our workouts, he and Cullen would banter back and forth about what they called 'The Countdown'. It was about when he would actually get the courage to seriously tell me how he felt about me."

"Do I need to say 'I told you so' again? He was crazy about you, from the start," Barb replied with a smile. "So, how are you holding up through all of it?"

"Honestly, I'm not. Everything about this makes absolutely no sense to me, Barb. How could I meet the most amazing man that's happened to my life and just when we're planning to fully and officially enjoy the joy of that, he dies?" I began to cry again for what felt like the hundredth time that day. "He died. He didn't breakup with me. He didn't stop texting or calling me. He didn't disappear only to appear with someone else on his arms later. He died! Although I know I still have so much to live for, including my Emmy, I feel like a part of me died with him also," I cried even harder.

"I'm so sorry Whit. It's so shocking and so devastating. From the moment you told me a couple of days ago, I still don't quite know what to say," Barb responded with complete compassion as she came across the kitchen island to hug me more than I could even explain that I needed.

"What's there to say?" I responded with far more helplessness than haughtiness as I allowed my head to collapse on her shoulder. "It's so outrageous. So ridiculous. So unbelievable. I keep waiting for my phone to ring and someone, anyone to tell me that this has been a huge mistake, a huge joke. And then, Cory comes running out from behind a huge curtain with his huge smile and one of his goofy dances to tell me it's all okay because he's actually okay. But, that's never going to happen because... he's never coming back," I continued with deeper sobs. "Death is... final. His death... is final. There's no do overs. There's no... second chances. There isn't a huge curtain or a trap door that he's waiting to peek out of. Yet, I feel trapped in so many emotions. All these emotions that don't explain the half of how deeply I'm hurting as I long for him and still love him as if he's right here."

"Is there anything I can do? Anything? Do I need to help with Emmy?" Barb asked as she hugged me closer while I let out more sobs.

"No, not really. I think by the time she gets home this afternoon, I'll be all out of tears for at least a couple of days," I responded as I tried to regain my composure. "As much of a mess I've been, I really miss her. Julian offered to keep her with him until the rest of the week, but I haven't seen her since Saturday morning. Although I told her the main details of what's going on over the phone yesterday, I don't want her to worry about me or think she's not a priority to me beyond all of this."

"Emmy knows you care about her. She also knows how much you cared about Cory. She won't expect you to be okay overnight She's a kid, but you raised a pretty smart kid," Barb assured me in the big sister voice she often used to remind me I wasn't the only strong one of the both of us. "Just don't try to be supermom in all of this, Whit. You've got to give your heart some time to heal before you start trying to prove to Emmy, or anyone that you're okay. Have you even considered my suggestion to make an appointment with Dr. Lansing pretty soon? It will definitely help you to talk to a professional, and you've always said she was incredibly helpful during the aftermath of your divorce?"

"Yes, I've thought about it. However, setting up a session with her would be such a huge reminder of who I was before I made all the decisions to allow my life to get better after connecting with Cory. If you remember, I stopped seeing her pretty much the same week I started working out with him. I think she was more relieved than I was that I was moving on. I gave her so much hell at times," I chuckled, realizing how much life had changed when Cory had officially came into my life.

The realization of how I would have to deal with life without him brought another wave of overwhelming frustration and fear to my exhausted heart all over again. I hadn't eaten consistently since Sabrina had delivered the news to me on Saturday morning. I hadn't worked out at the gym or at home, and I couldn't imagine having the energy to workout anytime soon. Most of my energy was spent trying to gather the energy to stop the tears which seem to flow more than I thought humanly possible. My only physical activity had been from mostly picking up my phone to either make sure I contacted everyone who needed to know the details of what was going on, or to respond to those who were constantly making sure I was continually going on.

Olivia cried almost as deeply as I had upon hearing the news. Kristina not only offered multiple prayers and encouragement, but she also made it clear that everyone at Radiant Reveals would fully support my decision to take a brief leave of absence instead of just the few days off I'd requested. Julian responded with a deeper state of understanding and remorse than I would've ever expected from him. Mom called with kind words that made me think someone had actually inhabited her body and downloaded specifically helpful words for her to say. She not only told me how sorry she was to hear about my loss but also how much she'd be willing to share with me some of the materials that helped her to deal with the aftermath of losing dad.

As bright as the lights of encouragement and offers of help shone round about me, the darkness of the loneliness and aching of my soul was overwhelming. My heart was ripped to shreds, as the man I loved had been ripped from my life. The reality of the tragedy was as thick as my tears were heavy. No matter how much I let the fountains of tears flow and then mustered the strength to turn it all off again, I felt shattered. My heart hurt more deeply than it had been filled with love and excitement just days before. The excitement of a love I'd never expected to find again was replaced with a wretchedness I'd never expected to feel, only moments after the bliss of it all had settled in. I felt as if life had dangled a shiny carrot before me of indescribable love and hope, only to destroy it midair as I reached out with delight to claim and enjoy my treasure. Even more, the saddest part of all my sadness was I no longer felt my heart could ever trust the feelings of complete happiness again.

"Mom, are we having pizza again tonight?" Emily whined.

"Yes, we are. And yes, I made sure your favorite pineapple topping is on both sides of it," I responded with a tone I hoped made an unofficial announcement to her that I didn't want to discuss much more about it.

"Well, I know you used to only let me have pizza on Thursday nights, but we had it on Monday, and now we're having it again today, and we had it like three times last week," she moaned a bit while trying to muster up a way to state the obvious. "Are we not eating the stuff we were eating before anymore? I mean, I'm not in love with asparagus and chicken, and brown rice and kale, and all that other stuff you have on your lists in your training folder. It just seems like you're doing everything so different now since... since... you know. Since Cory's not here anymore."

It had been six weeks and four days since my heart had been ripped to shreds by the news that the love of my life would no longer be in my life, as his life had been abruptly taken in a very random and ridiculous accident. As much as I knew it would certainly honor the amazing memories of Cory for me to have just pressed on and continue the fit lifestyle he had passionately taught me how to live, I didn't have the desire or drive to do anything beyond barely making it through my work schedule and returning home to be as alert of a mom as I could be to Emily.

I knew I wasn't dealing incredibly well at all, and I wasn't all too apprehensive about it being so apparent to those who were informally watching out for my life's details. My heart had been shattered in pieces, and I wasn't interested in hearing loads of useless advice on how to cope with the fragments when I had no hope that there would ever be full restoration. Although I knew it could definitely help to start working out again, I was no longer open to working off my stress in a manner which only reminded me of everything I had lost even after the joy of having lost so much weight.

Thus, I battled much of the battle with every comfort food I could get my hands on. The bulge was beginning to come back fully to my waistline as I ate whatever I wanted whenever I wanted. In fact, eating was all I seemed to want to do when I wasn't able to lullaby myself to sleep with rounds of tears from the tons of frustrated emotions that flowed with every tear.

Although my body had initially fought hard to process the poison I was pumping into it when I first returned to my binges of oversized cheat meals with huge bowls of desserts and piles of snacks, my new routine was in place. I was eating more garbage than I had actually remembered giving up before. Barb and Olivia were unbelievably understanding when they'd first caught wind of the new behavior of my old habits. Even so, their constant invitations to join them for our formerly fun workouts at the gym had soon become more frustrating than my waiting endlessly in the drive thru line for a crappy burger. My only moments of success was when I decided that some dairy cravings weren't worth the rumblings of a gaseous stomach keeping me up at night; I preferred my grieving tears be the cause of my sleeplessness and irritable bowels.

It was more and more evident that I'd tossed most every promise I'd made to myself of staying committed to the lifestyle I'd once worked so hard to maintain and enjoy. I could no longer drive pass Dynamo Fitness, much less go in for a workout, and I wanted nothing to do with my bright and cheery exercise room at home. Albeit, the thought that Cory could very well be turning over in his grave as I trampled all over everything he had instilled in me was more than I could bear at times.

I had already gained back over 20 pounds, and I was steadily pushing towards more. Yet, that wasn't the hugest of all my huge frustrations. I was cheekily irritated about the fact that my body's digestive system was nauseously rejecting the breads and pastries I was determined to add back to my daily meals of comfort. And to add insult to all the injury I was pouring upon my body, I was incredibly disappointed that I could no longer fit into quite of a few of the outfits I'd bought during my period of losing weight and feeling absolutely great. Nonetheless, the grief I felt in my heart and soul left me no solid energy to alter any of the imbecile behavior I had taken up once again.

"No, he's not here anymore, Emmy. But even if Cory were here, I'd still have a slice of pizza or two with you," I blatantly lied to her as if she hadn't watched the details of my life and habits just over a month ago.

"That's so not true, Mom. You weren't even buying real potato chips anymore when Cory was here. Now all we eat is Cheetos and Doritos with pretty much everything," she responded with more truth than tenacity in her voice.

"So, you were complaining about all the healthy food months ago, Emmy, and now you're still complaining. Your favorite pizza is right here on the counter, and every potato chip and snack you can imagine is in the pantry. The fridge is also packed with everything that could be placed on your personal list of favorite foods, yet you're still unhappy," I responded with as much exhaustion as there was embarrassment in my voice.

"I'm not unhappy, Mom. I'm just wondering. I'm just asking because everything is so different again." She responded with a slight confusion in her voice that I didn't really care to get to the bottom of just then.

"Well, until you become responsible for the crazy schedule it takes to run this home, how about you keep some of your insightful thoughts and questions to yourself, young lady?" I shot back with no attempt to hide the frustration in my voice.

"Mom, I didn't mean to make you angry. You were just doing so good with all your fitness stuff for so long. Now, everything is different. Everything. We're eating the stuff you swore we wouldn't ever buy again just weeks ago, and you don't ever go to the gym anymore," she replied while trying her best to keep a strong voice without the whining she knew I seriously couldn't stand when I was exhausted or annoyed or both. "I'm only mentioning it because you were so much happier before. I mean you barely smile at me now, unless you suddenly realize that I'm realizing that you're just not smiling at all."

"Yes, everything is different Emmy. I wish I could explain it all to you, but I can't right now because I can't quite explain it to myself. I wish I could just make you feel wonderful 24 hours a day as I continuously smile at you," I reacted with complete surrender and sarcasm in my tone. "I wish I could figure out exactly what to feed you and when to feed it to you, and what mood of yours will most enjoy what type of food we eat on what day. Even more, I guess it's not enough that your supermom is already trying to figure out how to throw a super birthday party for you next month despite all the craziness of everything going on, and despite the fact that I completely overlooked my own birthday just last week."

"Mom, that's not what I was saying at all. I was just asking because I'm worried about you, especially since you never ignore your birthday. Almost everyone in North Dallas knows that July 11th is just as huge to you as the 4th of July, which we didn't do anything huge for. That's why I'm worried about you. I'm not worried about me. I'll be okay. And, I'll be totally okay without having a birthday party because it only ends up being a reunion for all the grown-ups anyway. It's a huge festival of everyone trying to compare the presents that everyone bought for me," she explained with her way too grown up persona. "I know how to deal with you being unhappy, and Dad being annoyed at everything right now. It just bothers me because you guys think you can't talk to me about stuff."

"What does Dad have to do with this? What are you talking about, Emmy?" I insisted to understand her statement which I knew was her attempt to possibly reveal so much I'd obviously missed during such a time of grief.

"You're unhappy all the time, and Dad is always angry. Mom, every single day you look like you want to go downtown and jump off of a building. I think the only reason you don't do it is because you're maybe afraid of what would happen with me. The only time you don't look like you're going to start crying all over again, as if I don't know that you cry all the time, is when you're eating," she continued on with a completely respectful tone void of all fear, as if she'd been holding her words inside for ages. "You're eating all the stuff you promised to never eat again when Cory's whole notebook of everything was pretty much the bible to you. I know that you're unhappy mom, but it just makes me unhappy to see how you're not even trying to be happy again, at all. Then, I have to go to Dad's and deal with him being angry because he and Miss Karen are always mad at each other now, all the time."

"What? What are you talking about, Emmy? They're planning a wedding, sweetie. It's probably really stressful for them." I honed in on what she mentioned about Julian and Karen, as I had no energy to discuss the obvious she had obviously been observing about me.

"It's so much more than that, Mom, but I haven't said anything to you about it because I know you already have enough on your mind trying to keep Cory's death off of your mind," she replied far too matter-of-fact y.

"Sweetheart, I'm sorry I haven't been myself lately, but you don't have to worry about me. I'll get through this, and I'm so sorry I've let you take on the job of taking on my worries, or Dad's worries. I'm so sorry. What's going on, Emmy?" I pressed on for full disclosure with an apologetic tone filled with as much guilt as the remorse I felt for her frustration.

"Well, it actually started when he and Miss Karen cancelled their trip the same weekend Cory died in that accident. Dad called off that trip because Karen had refused to sign some prenatural papers," she blurted out as if a huge weight had been lifted off of her entire body.

"Prenatural papers? What are prenatural... who told you..." I stammered a bit, trying hard to understand what she was trying to tell me.

"You know, Mom," she interjected. "The papers some couples sign before they get married, so that the other person doesn't take all of their money if they ever get a divorce," she explained with fully expressive emotions on her face and with her hands as if she were pushing through a tough moment in a game of charades.

"Oh, wow. No, it's prenup papers. It's called a prenuptial agreement, sweetheart," I blurted back to her although I was revealing the jolt of the news more to myself than to her. "How do you know... who told you that... who talked to you about this?" I stammered.

"Dad doesn't even know I know anything about it actually. He and I hung out that weekend by ourselves because Miss Karen went to visit some friends after they cancelled the trip. She called him that Sunday night to say she was staying a few days longer. Although he was arguing on the phone with her in his office, I could hear a lot of what he was saying to her because he was talking so loud. He was pretty much yelling," she continued on, trying to fully recall everything. "He was telling her she could pout and threaten him all she wanted, but he wasn't going to marry anyone without protecting himself and everyone involved. Especially since he has a child to consider no matter what," she grinned while revealing that statement. "Is Dad rich, Mom? Does he have a lot of money?"

"He works very hard, and he does well for himself. And for you, Emmy. We both do. And, he's right. You've always been his hugest priority, so I can understand his making sure their decision to marry doesn't negatively affect that in any way." I confirmed to her in the most non-biased voice I could gather in response to all she'd revealed to me. "Wow, I had no idea this was going on."

"I know. I didn't think you would want me to bother you with all of it, especially with everything else you're already dealing with," she tried to explain as if she were my big sister rather than my big girl who was clearly growing up way too fast. "It's just sort of crazy now because they don't talk about the wedding anymore, and I know she was supposed to do a lot of stuff with me during the summer to get ready for it, but it's almost August already. I don't ask because they're both always aggravated at each other, and they aren't even good at hiding it. We don't eat dinner in the kitchen together anymore. Dad and I go to the living room most of the time, and Miss Karen always goes to her office or in the sunroom. She's still nice to me, but she just doesn't say much."

"Well, I'm really sorry to hear that. No matter what I think about your Dad and Karen being together, it's never easy to go through a tough time in a relationship. I hope they can somehow figure it out. It's worth it to try to make love work if we can. Then again, tomorrow isn't promised, and a happy heart isn't final." I responded matter-of-factly as my new-found views of cynicism resurfaced to reveal every bit of the unhappiness residing in my heart.

CHAPTER TWELVE

Broken Crayons Still Color

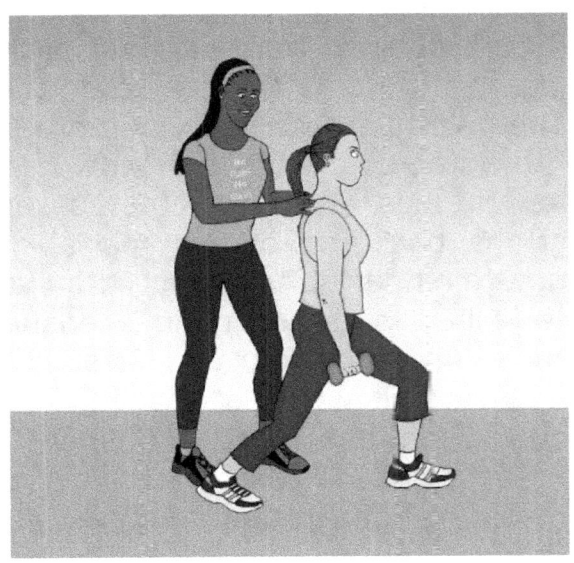

"Can you believe our baby girl is already 12 years old now?" Julian grinned, beaming at Emmy as she opened her new iPad while squealing multiple rounds of thanks to everyone for giving her so many cool gifts at her pool party packed with mounds of her friends and family standing in celebration of her.

Barb and Rick's manicured backyard was the perfect backdrop for the birthday extravaganzas Julian and I continued to throw for her every year since our divorce. Their massive stucco home boasted an outdoor patio with a state of the art kitchen and oversized underground pool that was as equally ornate as the Tuscan themed rooms throughout their home's interior.

We'd both decided from her first birthday that over the top was the only thing we'd do for Emmy's birthday. The pact had become even more significant as we'd both agreed we wouldn't throw her party at either of our homes after our divorce. We simply didn't want the backdrop of her special day to be another huge reminder of how much the dynamics of her family life had changed, ensuring our commitment to giving her our odd version of a great childhood. Whether it was a scavenger hunt, a tea-party, or the posh pool party I'd spent the past month precisely planning past every bit of the pain I was determined to fight through, Emily's big day was always a big deal to us.

"When she's acting like she's 25 years old, yes I can. But, when she's moaning and whining like the 2-year-old who didn't behave well for either one of us, no I can't." I laughed, almost tearing up at how proud I was of what Julian and I had built in Emily even though we ourselves were still undone in so many areas. I had no doubt she was the best thing that had happened to us, despite the worst of times having occurred between us.

"So, how are you doing overall?" He asked in a tone far too sincere to ignore.

Julian found every opportunity to chat with me at the party. Karen clearly hadn't attended with him though he'd shared her regrets for not being able to join us. He said it was due to a meeting with a photographer for her couture blog that just couldn't be rescheduled. She'd been supposedly waiting for weeks to connect with the individual's in demand schedule. Albeit, the expressions on Julian's face had never been good at concealing the truth, and the fact Emily had already told me way too much about what he had no idea we both knew, told me everything I needed to know: everything I completely understood he wasn't okay to tell me, or anyone right then and there.

"I'm much better than I was weeks ago. I'm not back to 100 percent for sure, yet I'm not running completely on empty anymore. I've also started working out consistently again," I replied with a real smile.

Though it was incredibly tough to be at Emily's pool party which I had eagerly looked forward to months before when my body had looked and felt better than it had in years, I stood rather tall as I chatted with Julian. While I was wearing a few of the overall 30 pounds I'd piled back on after Cory's death, I wasn't wearing the guilt or shame of having regressed in my goals, especially as I considered how hard I'd worked over the past few weeks in order to get some of the returned weight off.

I'd somehow peeled myself off the couch and out of my pile of tear-stained pillows to get back into working out at home. As much as I longed to go back to every bell and whistle I'd left with my membership privileges at Dynamo Fitness, I knew it would pull more motivation from me to force myself back into that beautiful building anytime soon. The motivation I'd already fought to muster up just to get moving again was precious to me, and I wouldn't poison it by dragging it through an atmosphere sure to cause me more heart wrenching pain.

I'd lost about 14 pounds as I'd consistently begun to eat clean again and work with the numerous methods I'd learned from Cory. The equipment I'd gathered at home over the years of starting and stopping and starting my journey all over again proved for good use again. The more I pushed through every tough rep of everything so tough to even think about doing, the more I recalled how important it was to push my mind to propel my body to move like my life was worth rebuilding—a rebuilding that would happen even if I couldn't find every broken piece and put it perfectly back together all at once.

As bored out of my mind as I was in working out solo, it felt so much better than mindlessly eating the crap which everything inside of me had no longer wanted. I'd sat on my ass for too long as my body longed to move and live with the energy it had enjoyed for months until my miserable sabbatical of grief. Nonetheless, as tough as I fought to get my life back, the fight was incredibly tough to fight through. There were times I lay curled up on my workout mat in a ball of involuntary tears as I sorely missed Cory's voice. I deeply missed his motivation and merriment that powered me through everything I struggled to maintain the power and proper form to do. Even so, I kept moving and believing I really could keep moving if I simply chose to.

I can't quite explain how I got through every tough moment. Maybe it was because I allowed myself to ponder upon the positive spirit and energy he'd always brought to everything we did. Maybe it was because of my choosing not to focus on the pain of losing Cory's strength, but to recall how much he'd always reminded me of everything I could do no matter how weak I felt in that moment. Or, maybe it was because I was done with feeing sorry for my sorrow which I somehow realized was only to make me stronger than I'd ever been through every weakness.

Every pushup felt as if I'd never get my body off the ground again, and every plank felt as if I was dying on the inside as I grieved the loss of him and the loss of progress I'd lost in the grieving process. Albeit, I somehow pushed on. Every jump squat, and burpee slam, and jackknife crunch felt more awful in my solo workouts than they'd ever felt when Cory had barked the reps out to me. Nonetheless, I had no doubt the quality of my life depended upon pushing forward to continue on taking control of my life and health in the way he'd taught me how: one crazy rep at a time. Choice by choice, I continued to revamp my mind as I pushed my body to gain back life, despite my overwhelming grief of experiencing the loss of such an amazing life.

"That's so good to hear," Julian replied. "Nothing about everything you've experienced over the past couple of months has been easy, Whit. To see how you're still holding it all together and all the while making sure our baby girl is okay says a lot about how good of a baby mama I chose," he laughed out loud at the facetiousness of his statement.

"Yes, you did pick a good baby mama, because you're wise. A wise ass, but wise indeed," I laughed deeper than I had in quite some time since the pain that had engulfed my heart. "Julian, you knew when you saw me in that student center years ago that the happiness of your life depended upon wisely inviting me to be a part of your life. Who knows? You could've been the dad of a really dense or hideous looking kid right now if it weren't for me," I continued with a facetious chuckle. "Speaking of happiness and wisdom, how's your next nuptial plans going? Are you and Karen ready to take over Hawaii?"

"Well, I hate to admit this to the face that may laugh out loud in my face up on hearing it, but our wedding plans are not really going at the moment," he confessed with what seemed like an odd sense of relief in his voice.

"What? What are you saying?" I tried my damnedest to seem far more surprised than he seemed embarrassed to share the truth of what I'd already known and sensed for weeks since Emily had shared her awareness of it all.

"It's a long story with my short version of it, but it is what it is," he began. "I made the assumption she would totally understand why I wouldn't want to go into a marriage without a prenup after we've both failed at marriage once before. Although she and I were mostly solid over the past few years, we didn't start our relationship on solid ground," he continued on, talking more to himself than to me while gathering his words. "The fact that I have to protect my ability to always provide fully for Emmy makes a prenup closed for demonstrative debates, with or without expensive lawyers. We've tried to work past it, but it's all or nothing for her. I simply won't grant her the opportunity to take everything she can from me if we ultimately don't work out. She was shafted financially by her ex-husband, and I really sense she's trying to score big with me," he grimaced at his thoughts while continuing on. "We haven't officially called off the wedding, yet we haven't continued planning any aspects of it either. Plus, now that we're mostly sleeping in separate rooms unless Emmy's at the house, I think we both know what the next chess move is, even if we both feel like pawns in the grand scheme of it all."

"Julian, I don't really know what to say. I can imagine you're not feeling too great about any of this. So, I really am sorry about that." I replied as honestly I could. I had no remorse in things not working out between him and the woman I knew had carefully calculated her plan to finish off the destruction of our marriage from the day I'd invited and trusted her into our lives.

"I actually thought you would've gotten a good laugh about it. Maybe you can include in your order of black roses for us a condolence card, instead of congratulations this time?" He forced a funny, acknowledging I had full opportunity and reason to gloat at the revelation of such news.

"Ha-ha! Yes, the black roses," I laughed out loud, recalling the rude statement I'd made to him months before when we'd discussed him and Karen's engagement. "Every good laugh does help me these days, Julian. However, I've been through enough pain myself not to enjoy watching anyone else having to go through a tough time, especially when it comes to matters of the heart."

"I know you don't wish any malice towards me, Whit. It is tough though realizing you'll have your grand opportunity to say I told you so pretty soon," he replied with more defeat than I'd heard in his voice in quite some time. "It's not just that things have been awful since all the arguing about the prenup; it's just that a few other things haven't been adding up also, for quite some time. I think, well I actually know, she's seeing someone else. I don't even have interest in really getting to the bottom of the whole story with her. It's our friend who she was dating before her and I got involved, Ian. I should've seen it coming, but everything happens for a reason."

"Ian? I'm so sorry, Julian." I gasped a bit. "That has to be devastating to come back full circle like that. And yes, a year or so ago I probably would've river danced at hearing something like this, but your baby mama is far more healthier and mature, physically and mentally row," I chuckled a bit, attempting to lighten the heavy burden displayed all through his words and face.

"I'm actually somewhat glad about all of it though. When I make my decision this weekend, I won't feel awful in thinking she has nowhere to go," he responded with far more resolve than emotion. "I already have a small settlement prepared for her so we can break ties fully. I have no doubt she'll require some sort of compensation as we've been together in common law for a few years now."

"So, you've already made a decision about this. When do you plan to tell Emmy about it?" I asked him in a slight mama bear tone.

"Well, I think she may already have an idea of what's going on, but I'm planning to officially tell her everything in the next couple of days. I definitely don't want to ruin her birthday celebration week. Then again, this may the best gift ever for her," he laughed, locking eyes with my expression which didn't hide my own humor in his statement. "She was never a huge fan of Karen, and we both know she wasn't all too excited about the wedding."

"Julian, I seriously don't know what to say. I feel like it was just moments ago I was figuring out how to even deal with the news of you deciding to officially marry her," I replied with a sincerity and compassion in my voice I was sure caught us both by surprise. "Then moments later, I'm building a love that helped me forget the pain of any love I felt I'd lost before, only to seconds later experience the unbearable pain of losing all of that. Now, I'm hearing of the pain that's ahead for you in having to start all over again. This... this entire year seems to have had more life experiences packed into it than all the years we've all been alive," I forced a slight smile, biting back tears I knew could fall at any moment.

"It has been quite a year. But, who knows? It's only August, and a lot more good can come out of it. Truth is, we can't deny that a lot of good has already happened through all of it, despite the pain. Whit, we actually talk to each other now, with more respect than we probably both ever expected to have for one another again. We seriously listen to each other, with understanding beyond our own points of view," he continued on with a genuine smile of hope. "Who knows? We could end up rekindling our flame all over again. I know you couldn't possibly imagine anything like that right now with everything that's happened over the past few months, much less the past few years. I could totally see us back together one day though, if our stars are ever lucky enough," he grinned widely as he finished.

"A flame. What flame? Julian, you'd better count your lucky stars that I'm finally at a place where I don't want to set flames to your ass anymore, much less imagine us together in complete bliss again," I laughed out loud in complete mockery of his heartfelt words despite the fact the thoughts of my heart almost immediately whispered he'd probably be the one getting the last laugh in all of it.

"Never say never, Whitty! I've seen how you've been looking at me all day," he laughed as he and I chuckled at his sly choice of using his specific nickname for me.

"I didn't say never, Juju." I shot back as he grinned from ear to ear at my calling him the name I hadn't used since we last remembered truly being happy together. "But, I can't say my heart would be totally excited to completely open up to the man who once broke it into more pieces than I would've ever imagined."

"I can understand that," he smiled with an expression of complete empathy as his brown eyes seemed to glisten. "Just like I know you understand I'm not that same selfish man, and you're clearly not that same broken woman. Time will tell though."

"Well, until then I hope time tells you how impressed I am at your overall decision in all of this. It makes me happy to know you'll always decide what's best for Emmy," I smiled up at him with a heart that couldn't quite explain the compassion I felt for him.

"Thank you. I'm glad you're impressed. And, you should be even more impressed that I haven't listened at all to my urge to slap you on your seriously firm ass all afternoon. Your hard work is definitely working for you, Whitty," he laughed facetiously as we both smiled at the fact that absolutely everything, yet nothing at all had changed between us.

"I can't believe I put up with your insane ass kicking, yet I am so happy to be working with you, lady!" I smiled at Sabrina, trying to regain my breath and overall composure after another set of lunges. "It's unbelievable what you're able to do to my body while teaching me to convince my mind that it really enjoys the torture."

"Oh stop that bellyaching, Whit. You and I know you'd be more disappointed if my workouts pat your back instead of completely kicked your ass," Sabrina laughed. "Grab your mat so we can get your plank work in today."

"Aye, aye! Sergeant Psycho!" I teased as I grabbed my mat that was leaning on the light blue wall of her studio. The soothing light blue and chocolate brown color scheme of Sabrina's studio portrayed an oxymoron of the electric atmosphere she created in her pristine building. Even though her studio had far more space than equipment surrounding us, her sessions left my body feeling sorer than if I'd been elsewhere doing supersets all day long with every combination of workout tools imaginable. Her combinations of push-ups and plank work were as evil as they were effective. Even more, her strength based cardio blasting workouts, rarely requiring the use of anything outside of my own bodyweight, pushed me past every limit I attempted to place on myself. Just to be able to speak in full sentences after Sabrina's sessions was always a huge win for me, and apparently any of her clients I chatted with outside of our amazing time with her.

Sabrina's tiny frame boasted a tremendously huge smile which wasn't the typical build or persona I'd seen demonstrated amongst what some would consider a standard personal trainer. She was a dynamic individual who compelled individuals to look completely past her pretty girl looks to embrace her passion for life and health which was solidified by the fact she was clearly her own best client. Sabrina was as powerful as she was petite, and she was as energetic as she was enthusiastic. Her enthusiasm ran deep about coaching everyone under her tutelage on how to live their lives full of the life and energy she believed almost everyone desperately craved and deserved. Her incredibly toned 5′ 3″ frame, carrying barely 110 pounds. encompassed a personality that was as bright as her ebony skin was brown. Her passion and positivity had the consistency of her workout programs which were always filled with challenging sets of intensity, inspiration, and actual fun.

"I'm glad you're working with me too, Whit. It's really an honor considering how we were brought together in the first place," she continued smiling at me with the empathetic glance we often exchanged. It was a glance saying everything yet nothing about the huge loss we both still felt in losing the very significant yet very different bond we had both had with Cory. "And besides, you and I know you'll never get the butt you really want by sitting on the one you have. Albeit, you did a hell of a job on your own getting those pounds off that you'd piled back on," she smiled with admiration.

Though I had spent the past couple of months toughing out the process of getting my body back in action by working out solo at home, I knew it was time to go to the next level when I reached out to Sabrina. Going through the plethora of workouts I'd gathered from my time with Cory garnered good results for me; nevertheless, I headed her way knowing that being a part of the crazy action she'd continually grown at her studio could offer me the comradery and support that simply wasn't found at home in my personal workout room. I wanted a true mentor in my life again to set my ass on fire, and help me burn through the next levels in my fitness journey like never before.

Initially, it was a tough call to make considering the complexity of our history. Sabrina had lost one of the greatest friends and advisors of her life, and I'd lost the man who was very well becoming the love of my life, before he lost his life. The fact we were both getting on with life in spite of losing Cory furnished a bond between her and I that felt nothing short of a solid sisterhood.

"Yeah, I'm pretty glad to finally be back to the point I was at right before we lost him. Well, I'm actually in a size 10 now. I was in a size 12 when he and I transitioned our training and our relationship," I smiled on, attempting to accurately line up the heartfelt memories and details of my journey. "It feels like a new brand of punishment fully getting back at it though. Then again, I deserve the punishment for what I did to my body all over again after losing him," I smiled weakly confirming what I just knew Sabrina thought about the roller-coaster mode I'd taken again after Cory's death.

"You deserve punishment? Where did you get that avenue of thinking? Whit, you don't deserve punishment," she chuckled with disbelief. "You honestly deserve a good thump across the head for thinking punishment is what you deserve for being an imperfect human being who will never do everything perfect in your fitness journey, even if you're passionately committed to the process without any crazy interruptions," she smiled directly at me with a full sincerity. "You went through complete emotional and mental hell in losing Cory. Punishing yourself for having a complete collapse is as crazy as anyone possibly thinking you should be completely over the pain of losing a loved one in just a few months, or even a few decades."

"It was hell. It's still tough at times, although you know I've begun to move forward in a direction I had no thought I'd ever be going again," I smiled, thinking about the irony of how Julian and I's hearts had become reconnected in such a way that had surprised everyone around us. "And thank you for saying something so powerful like that. I know I'm in such a better place now, but you have no idea how much I've seriously beat myself up over quitting on myself, Sabrina. Especially after having accomplished so much in working with Cory. I just felt like I trampled all over the triumphs he and I had accomplished together when I failed to continue on after his death."

"He died, Whit, suddenly and tragically. A part of you probably died too, as you grieved the loss of him. To see everything you did or didn't do afterwards as completely failing isn't true. It isn't true at all. Failure isn't in falling down, ever. It's in refusing to ever get up again. You've not only gotten up, you're finding happiness and love in such a way again that only proves how much your heart and your life has healed and grown so much over the past year alone," she responded with as much intensity and compassion in her voice as was in her eyes. "I'm so happy for you and Julian."

"Thank you. I am too. I would've never thought he'd be a huge part of my healing and realizing life can go on again. The man who I'd once deemed a complete devil has actually become an incredible angel in my life all over again," I beamed.

"That's awesome," she replied while grabbing a few other pieces of equipment to continue my workout session. "I'm so happy to know how happy you are now. You were broken, Whit, so broken. All of us who mourned Cory's death felt so in some way or another. But, broken crayons still color. Sometimes even more vividly if we're truly determined to finish the project at hand."

"Broken crayons still color? That's powerful," I beamed, fighting not to tear up at the magnitude of what those words meant to me. "Where did you get that? Where do you get the crazy wisdom you share with me?"

"Ha-ha! I've tried to tell you that I read as much as I talk," she laughed, trying not to show embarrassment at my compliment to her. "Seriously, I told you Cory would always remind me if I want be an effective leader tomorrow, I have to decide wisely what I'm reading today. And, if I choose not to read anything much at all, I'm ultimately choosing not to lead anyone, at least not effectively. A reader today makes a leader tomorrow."

"You're absolutely right. My career certainly wouldn't be where it's at today if I didn't keep my nose in medical journals as often as I do," I agreed. "My psychiatrist mentioned I should probably pick up something new on parenting, and relationships in this new season for Julian and me. And of course on what I'm still experiencing in losing Cory. Even though I've moved on, the grief still stings."

"I can imagine so," she responded with a warm smile. "Something I learned in losing Cory is when we understand that death is ultimately a part of the life process, although a tragic part, we can focus on what really matters even more in our own lives as we courageously choose to go on with life. As tough as it is to focus on much of anything when we go through the pain of losing someone, it really is a good time to refocus on everything."

"Oh, God! Are we still talking fitness or are we doing grief counseling now?" I laughed in awe of her insight. "You've almost repeated some of the things verbatim that my psychiatrist just mentioned to me a couple of weeks ago. The patient declines to listen further, Dr. Sabrina."

"Oh, don't even try to play your sarcasm route with me, Whit," she laughed pretending to throw a dumbbell at me. "You know I'm not even close to being a professional counselor, although I should start charging you by the hour for my insight. Really though, we're just chatting about the things that matter in your life right now as you decide to fully get your life back again."

"I know, and I appreciate that about you, Sabrina. I really like that you're just as committed to challenging my thought process and strengthening my mind as you are in seriously kicking my ass through your every set of your torture. I think you're even crazier than Cory was in some ways," I laughed with full gratitude in my heart.

"Ha-ha! Well, I've learned from some of the very best in fitness," she beamed, continuing on with as much excitement in her voice as she had at the start of our session. "In fact, I think a good thing for you to do in the next couple of days is to really ponder on why you're still deciding to do this, Whit?"

"Why? What do you mean by why?" I replied with a slight bit of annoyance, considering her question pretty preposterous as I prepared for our next round of exercises. I clearly hadn't reached my fitness goals yet, and I'd obviously been struggling to completely reach them solo before I began my training again with her. Why? 'Because Y comes before Z' was what I almost exclaimed in response to her crazy question. I knew my body could still look and feel even better, and I wasn't interested in giving myself any more excuses to not push through to my own personal finish line. I'd literally struggled back to 174 pounds, and I was officially wearing a size 10 and sometimes an 8 on my 5'4" frame for the first time in years. Albeit, the fight wasn't over for me yet.

"What's your WHY? It's as simple and as difficult a question as that," she smiled with complete confidence in the question she'd asked. "Why do you want to continue your fitness journey, Whit? Despite all your ups and downs and the absolute roller-coaster behavior you've explained to me you've always dealt with, what's your why? Especially as you've mentioned the punishment you still feel like your body is going through as you

231

continue to press on through all of it," she pressed on. "You know, one of the best professionals I've ever followed in fitness once said that unless we bring our why into every workout with us, most everything we do to transform our body in the process will actually feel like punishment. So, what's your why?"

"Oh, my WHY, meaning my absolute motivation," I responded with a bit more patience as I found clarity in her explanation. "Well, I've tossed about 30 pounds on and off my body since my tanking after Cory's death, and I want to totally get back in shape again and completely finish my goals!" I answered with what I felt was not only a strong answer but also an obvious one needing no further questioning of why.

"Oh, no. Don't even think about stating the obvious, my friend," she retorted with her signature smile, waiting patiently for another response from me while I planked until my torso felt too numb to grasp the actual torture it felt. "We all want to get in shape. We all want to look good. We all want to obtain all the image related crap that amounts to much of nothing in our exhausted minds when the going gets tough as hell."

"Okay, I can agree with that," I laughed at her ability to call bullshit on any bullshit. "Well, a huge why for me is being healthy for Emily, being an example and a true strength for her. I want her to know I care about her enough to care about myself," I acknowledged, realizing Emily had always been the why inside of every facet of any why I could ever have.

"That's pretty commendable, but it's still sort of stating the obvious. Most every parent that cares anything about their children desires to be their absolute best for them. Although Kyle and I aren't parents yet, I can imagine a lot of our decisions will be centered on our children when we have them; however, the fuel of our decisions must stem even beyond them," she persisted on. "With all due respect, Whit, when I first met you when Cory was alive you shared with me that Emily had been your biggest inspiration and motivation in pursuing your fitness goals. Yet, when you relinquished again this last time, the why factor about Emily didn't keep you from deciding to bail out for a bit. I'm certainly not rubbing your nose is that choice because I completely understand how hard everything was for you in going through such a devastating loss. However, being healthy for Emily didn't continue to motivate you to take care of you. Family is such a significant motivation, but your motivation has to be even beyond your family."

"I so get your point, and even your reasoning behind your point, Sabrina. But WHYYYYY are we even talking about why?" I questioned with complete annoyance at her digging for more than I felt able to explain in that moment. I felt far more irritation than inspiration as she touched a nerve in me which no one beyond my personal world had the nerve to delve into. I hated her for it, and I hated the fact

233

that I was hating her for it, knowing she was taking the right trek up the mountain of my struggles.

"WHY? Because I care enough about you, and not just the achievement of your goals, to seriously ask you why. And, because I know we all have a why, beyond any weight or image issue. Beyond any family or relational issue, or any other issue that may be the obvious in our personal scenario. Whit, if we don't know our own personal why, we definitely won't stay consistent in showing ourselves that we mean business in our fitness goals. Truth is, lots of people watch family members suffer and sometimes die prematurely from complications of diabetes, heart disease, or another lifestyle related issues, and that doesn't always motivate them to begin or continue on in their fitness goals. Even more, far too many parents are overweight now as they raise overweight kids, and that doesn't get them going or keep them going in getting fit and healthy," she continued with a fervent smile, confirming her purpose was to seriously help me whether I felt so or not.

"So, what are you saying?" I responded, looking up at her from my workout mat with as much frustration as the exhaustion I felt from our session which still wasn't quite over.

"What I'm saying is that I'd be a pretty crappy trainer to let you off the hook with your simple answers and pseudo-responses that you don't even believe anymore, Whit. Even if it makes you a bit frustrated with me, my goal is to get to the heart of

234

what motivates your heart in this journey," she smiled with her *I know exactly what you're thinking* look. "All you've done for so many years is give the answers and the responses you've thought would please everyone else while not really considering what you really want as you've allowed your health to stay in roller-coaster mode, Whit."

"You may be right," I agreed reluctantly with a half-smile.

"I know I'm right, Whit," she smiled back at me with her frustratingly warm compassion. "You've tried transforming your life before to please Julian, and now you guys are only back together again because you've both matured and realized that an amazing relationship is not about trying to force each other to be more like each other but rather becoming an even better version of who your partner initially fell for," she preached on. "You've tried getting the weight off to be an example to Emily. You've tried remaining steady in order to gain your mom's respect and acceptance. You've tried to get after your goals to keep up with your cousin Barb. You've tried to stay consistent because of Cory and the honor of his memory. It's all been well-meaning, but when are you going to figure out WHY you're doing it for yourself, Whit? When are you really going to accept yourself, and have complete respect for yourself, and seriously cheer yourself on? When? And WHY?"

"Okay, I clearly I get it," I responded with tears forming in my eyes as I sat up on my workout mat. "So my why is *my* why?"

"Yes. Even if it is connected to someone else, it's still personally yours, Whit. For example, even though my life's purpose and career is in health & fitness, that isn't my why for staying in shape. I'm a trainer with a plethora of great clients, but that isn't my ultimate reason for taking care of myself. My actual why is because I want to truly live while I'm alive. I don't want to drag ass through life, Whit. I want to really live with energy, and strength, and focus, and confidence, and peace of mind in knowing I'm taking care of the gift of life God's given to me, even if I may have just one more day to enjoy it. I want to really live, every day of my life. That's why I put up with the punishment of all the work I do to my body. That's my WHY."

"That's pretty awesome, Sabrina. I've just always had a different approach to why I'm trying to get fit and stay fit. I think I've honestly thought more on why I *should be* getting in shape far more than why I actually *want to*. I've almost always felt like I've been in a constant fight with the looming threat of an early death, especially with the long list of health issues threatening the longevity of my life when I was seriously obese earlier this year. Not to mention, the breast cancer scare I had a little over a year ago. It all seemed to heighten the fear instead of motivating me to make a lasting change," I continued on as even more awakening occurred in my soul. "Sabrina, I lost my dad when he was only 51 years old due to kidney failure brought on by complications of Type II diabetes. Even more, my favorite aunt, who was more of a mom to me than my own mom, passed away just last year from a heart attack at only 57 years old. Although I don't say it, and I try not to think too much about it, I don't want that to be me. I don't want to leave Emily sooner than I have to, simply because I'm not taking care of my health. Yet, even the fear of all of that doesn't really keep me going consistently, and it never has."

"Because fear doesn't bring life or lasting motivation. It doesn't help us make powerful choices in our lives. Fear is as good at motivating us in our fitness goals as diet sodas are effective at helping us to chisel our abs," she continued on with a good laugh and a solid smile confirming she sensed that the light bulb was coming on fully in my heart and soul. "Although the warnings of dying prematurely can be a good cause to get our attention to start taking care of our bodies or continuing doing the work of staying healthy and fit, we know tomorrow isn't promised to us even if we're in great health. Hell, we learned that all over again from losing Cory, didn't we? However, today and every day that's given to us can be completely kick ass if we're kicking ass in taking care of ourselves."

"So my WHY in my fitness goals is ultimately about my own personal life even if it's directly related to someone in my life?" I affirmed out loud more to myself rather than to Sabrina.

"Yes it is, and rarely does anyone think about it in these terms, Whit, especially women. We so often think considering ourselves first is the ultimate act of selfishness," she responded with as much resolution as emotion in her voice. "If you were sitting on a plane with a toddler, receiving instructions on how to help your little one in case of an emergency during that flight, you would be instructed to place your own oxygen mask on before you even attempt to carry out the task of securing his or her mask on. Why? Because you can't offer complete help and support to someone else until you yourself are fully taken care of. In the air or on the ground, it's you first or everyone else will ultimately hurt."

"Where do you get this stuff, woman? You're like an energetic ball of wisdom, and strength, and compassion, and hilarity, and physical pain all rolled into one," I laughed out loud realizing yet again how fortunate I was to have such a kick ass individual in my corner helping me to fight through everything that had continuously cornered me in the pursuit of my fitness goals.

"Whit, you are far more amazing than I am," she smiled admiringly at me. "Hello, just the fact you completed years of intense study and schooling to acquire the degrees and qualifications necessary to obtain the career you seriously rock at proves that you really don't have quitting ingrained into your

DNA. Nonetheless, you seem to think you're such a quitter when it comes to your fitness goals. Even more, you're raising a daughter who's more strong and remarkable than either of us were probably willing to be at her age. That says a lot about the wisdom you've poured into her, and the compassion you've done it with."

"That's quite a compliment. I wish I could consistently focus a bit more on what you see about me, and what so many others have seen," I smiled at her, admitting the mental cavities that were still evident in my journey. "I do try to focus on the good stuff much more than I ever have, but it's tough to do so when there's so many voices barking at me from my past mistakes and choices, and so many fears and worries blaring about my upcoming decisions and plans."

"I totally get it, Whit. Fear isn't always the issue that stops us either. So many of us simply set no great expectations of ourselves when it comes to pushing forward and accomplishing what we truly want," she continued with a fresh fire in her voice as if she hadn't already poured out rivers of wisdom to me all morning. "We don't always cower in fear. We also rule ourselves out of being strong, and able, and fierce, and downright awesome at so many things."

"Ok, I've got to ask you. How have you become who you are? I'm not talking about professionally. I already know your certifications, etc. I know you've said you didn't have an easy childhood, or even a great time as an adult up until just a few years ago. And, I know they didn't teach you the essence of who you are in 'personal trainer school'. Even in grad school I learned more about how to look after other people than how to take care of myself," I laughed out loud at the truth of my statement. "So, how are you so ridiculously awesome, Sabrina, and always ready to inspire others on how to get after it in life too?"

"Awesome? Well thank you, Whit, but flattery won't get you easier warm-ups or longer cool downs. And, it won't get you out of the rest of this workout. Okay?" She laughed as we set up for my final rounds of push-ups and plank work. "Really though, thank you. I think I mentioned to you in one of our first conversations that I'm really huge on affirmations. Daily affirmations. Talking to myself about myself as I become all I know I was created and purposed to be," she smiled with confidence, continuing on to explain. "At 35 years of age I've finally learned that if it's not positive, or powerful, or progressive, it can't continue to come out of my mouth. I'm also committed to doing the daily work it takes to keep the tons of garbage that can come in from so many sources out of my head. I've learned to be more in control of what's going on in my head, as that's what ultimately comes out of my mouth," she chuckled, playfully patting her head as she covered her mouth. "I stay aware of what I read, watch, and listen to. I understand it all filters in and through me. I read somewhere once that we must be careful how we are talking to ourselves because we are listening." She finished with a beaming smile.

"We must be careful…" I attempted in awe to repeat the words that made more sense to me than my senses could quite contain. "Say that again."

"We must be careful how we are talking to ourselves because we are listening," she repeated with a smile shining as bright in her voice as the one on her face. "We humans are notorious at berating and bashing ourselves, Whit. Especially we women, even in what we consider to be a playful manner. There's nothing ever funny about calling yourself a fat ass, ever. As tiny as I am, you won't hear me calling my 5'3", 110 pound frame a bag of bones, ever.

"You're so right! Cory used to always get after me for that!" I exclaimed with a smile, my heart flooding with good memories for a brief moment. "Even more, Barb has always reminded me of how powerful affirmations are. I've honestly thought she's so big on them because she's already so beautiful and powerful. Then again, I've had clients who are gorgeous on the outside, yet the overall negative attitude in their words radiate nothing pass their pretty faces," I acknowledged as another light bulb went off in my soul. "Even so, I've tried saying positive things out loud to myself before, but it doesn't feel natural to me."

"It's probably never going to feel completely natural if you don't practice it consistently, Whit. We live in a society so consumed by how we look on the

241

outside and who we long to please and impress it that. We've got to understand how important it is to take the time to focus on the impression we're ultimately making upon our own hearts and souls. We make that impression with our every word and every choice surrounding our words."

"Wow, that's a lot to digest," I smiled at her with an official thank you in my expression.

"Oh, you're welcome. You can tell Dr. Lansing I've clearly got her back," she teased. "By the way, you don't have to have the answer to your why immediately, nor do you have to share the depth of it with me. I do challenge you to get to the bottom line of it and why it's there though, Whit. I assure you it'll be one of your biggest wins as you push on towards every other victory. It'll also help you continue to get through every rough session I'll always have in store for you," she warned me with a good laugh.

"Oh, I know," I laughed out loud with her. "I actually think I already know it though, and you'll know it soon enough." I smiled inside out, feeling full gratitude again for being given yet another opportunity to get it right in my journey.

CHAPTER THIRTEEN

Feel Free to Call Me Whit

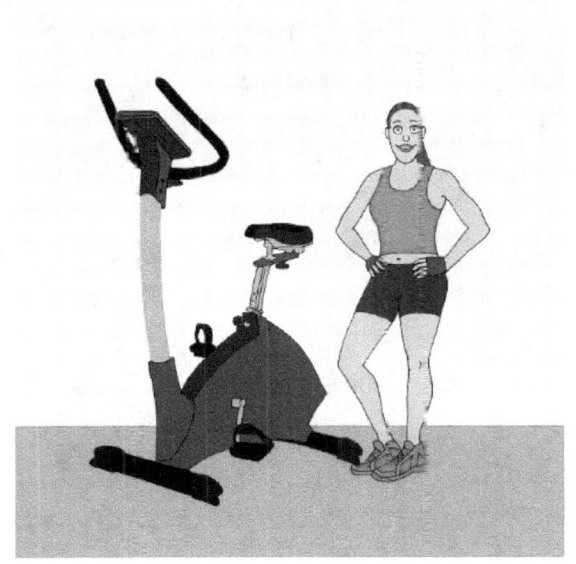

"**I** can't even begin to tell you how proud I am of you, Whit. Look at you. Everything about you is absolutely radiant inside out. You're beautiful. You're practically glowing," Mom smiled across the kitchen island at me with what seemed like full tears forming in her eyes. "And, to have things be so much better between us now means more to me than anything."

"Thank you, Mom. Thank you also for the strength you've been to me over the past few months. Like I told you before, from the moment you reached out to me after Cory died, I knew I should try to do everything I could to make sure we had a decent relationship again," I smiled back at her, taking in every moment of what we'd been experiencing in rebuilding a bond between us that'd never really been there before. "It certainly didn't feel good to hear the things you said to me months ago. Even so, I had to take a really good look at the dynamics of all of it, and understand why you could have a reason to have the viewpoint you had. It was awfully hard to hear, but I understand now where you were coming from."

"Well, it definitely wasn't all because of you, Whit. Even if it had been, I could've chosen a better way to say all of that to my own daughter," Mom confessed with a transparency in her voice that I hadn't even recalled from childhood. "Of course that revelation came by my taking an honest look at myself and finally getting some solid professional help. I didn't realize how long and how deeply I've grieved the loss of Dad. Even though I chose to put a completely different face on all of it, I've been hurting," she acknowledged. "I was so mad at him for so long for leaving us so soon. He left us all because of his mostly prideful and selfish choices to refuse to adhere to any of the warnings about his health, and it wounded me. He ignored even the very early on warnings, and it hurt to realize I was powerless to do anything about it. However, as much as we didn't get along during his last years here with us, I really loved your dad. Sweetheart, I was crazy about him from the day we met. I just felt so unappreciated, so disrespected, so betrayed as his health declined more and more. Then, after we lost my only sister last year, it just brought in a whole new wave of the hurt, loss, and regret I'd already been engulfed in for years," she finished.

"Mom, I seriously thought you hated me after Dad died. You would barely talk to me, unless I had Emmy with me. Then, when Aunt Catherine died last year, you and Barb became even closer. I just knew your heart was completely shut off to me," I revealed, trying my best to hold back the waterfall of tears attempting to move past the choking up that had begun in my throat.

"Are you kidding? I've never hated you, Whit. Although you were clearly Daddy's girl, you'll always be my baby girl, my only baby girl," she smiled as she explained further. "I did hate how much you seemed to proudly mimic Dad's habits, but I also hated that I never quite knew how to help you through all of it. I let so many years pass between us without reminding you of how much you mean to me and how devastated I'd be if I'd lost you. Even though I was too hurt and angry most of the time to have the energy to show it, I was very afraid of losing you for the same reasons we lost Dad. Sweetheart, I can't change anything about what happened years ago or even all that's happened in this year alone, but I do love you, and I really do believe we can ultimately decide how the rest of our story is written," she finished with a sincere smile, expressing more love than I'd seen in years on her face.

"I love you too, Mom. It has been quite a year for sure. I keep wishing that I'd kept a diary of some type, or at least a journal of the details of this entire year. I can recall all of the details of my physical changes of course. How can I not?" I laughed as we both smiled in awe of the obvious. "I'm 148 pounds, and I'm wearing a size 6 now. A size 6, Mom. I wasn't even in a size 6 when Emily was six years old. At the start of this year I was in a size 20 and pushing the scale completely past 250 pounds," I beamed with so much excitement and gratitude in my heart.

"That's over 100 pounds or so lost, Whit. With every high and low you've experienced, you've seriously pushed through and did the work to get such incredible results. Despite every setback you probably thought would shut you down altogether, you've just become a shining example of what happens when we press forward to make it happen. What you've done is amazing. Who you've become is amazing," she grinned as we both took in the power of the moment we shared.

"It is amazing. I can't believe how much of me has changed mentally and emotionally. It sure would be almost hilarious to be able go back and remember what was going on in my brain. Like when I first met Cory in January, or when I did the Fun Run with Emmy in the spring. Even when I went on my first shopping spree with Barb after I'd lost about 50 pounds. I had so many thoughts and emotions going on that weekend," I grinned at the memory of so many memories. "I did decide to start a journal right after Julian and I's first date not too long ago. September 18th. I actually called the entry 'As Happy As if Hell Never Happened'," I laughed out loud as Mom grinned from ear to ear at the sound of Julian and I being together again.

"Ha-ha! Well, I hope it's more heavenly this time around. Really though, you know I've always liked Julian with you, Whit. We all did. Even in the worst of times you guys went through, he was always really good to you. He's also such an amazing dad to Emmy, just as Juan was to you. I know you always felt like I took his side when you guys split up, but it broke my heart to see your marriage that was set up so well to succeed completely fail by simple yet serious negligence," she continued as she bit back tears again. "Julian put up with your behavior for a long time before he crumbled under the pressure of it all. That slimy Karen just came sliding in at the right time for all the wrong reasons. I know, I shouldn't be rehashing all of this," Mom finished with a faint smile.

"It's okay, Mom. I know you're not trying to hurt me or smear anything in my face. It's hard not to talk about all the history Julian and I have had together. We were just discussing the other night how the toughest thing for us is probably going to be in deciding which good memories to keep and which bad ones to bury forever if we're going to make awesome new memories. One of the best things about all of it is that we've really been open and honest with ourselves and to each other about where we know we really screwed it up before," I smiled, thinking about how good our new times together had already been. He and I were like the two college kids who had met years ago, learning everything about each other all over again. "I shared with him a quote I read recently on the internet that really hit me between the eyes. It opened my eyes even more to the damage I'd done to our relationship long before Karen came in to destroy the rest of it."

"What did it say?" Mom stared intently for an answer as if it her own life depended upon hearing it.

"Something like if we behave in a manner that brings poison into our relationship, we can't be surprised when it ultimately dies." I replied as the words reawakened me all over again. "It was hard to admit to myself and to Julian that our marriage ultimately crumbled because I wasn't the wife he needed or wanted for years. Julian adored everything about me, but no man adores insecurity or cruelness. And, he definitely can't handle a cute blend of the both of them when his every effort to make things better are being disregarded," I laughed to keep from tearing up at the memories of my behavior. "Although my weight was an issue between us, it wasn't the ultimate issue. It never was. You know, Mom, Julian had never really made my weight an issue until he saw how all the other issues going on in me was causing me to be totally okay with my weight rapidly increasing. And, when the health problems and scares that came with it surfaced, he really took a strong stance because he wanted his wife to be okay," I confessed without any shame in what my behavior of yesterday once destroyed.

"Wow, I am so proud of you, Whit. It's never easy to admit when we know we were wrong. And, to fully admit your wrongdoings with a solid apology says even more about who you are versus what you've done," she smiled at me with enough admiration to propel me through the rest of life itself.

"Well, I've got to get it right this time, Mom. He and I both do," I gleamed, looking forward in my mind's eye to the exciting days ahead. "Especially with Emmy being at an age where she completely understands our communication even without words. We've raised a pretty smart kid who has that only child slash unofficial grown up persona that works for us and against us."

"Yes, she's so much like you when you were her age, Whit. Albeit, you were far more dramatic,"

Mom laughed out loud as I gave her a *please don't go down memory lane* look. "Just don't take it personally if she takes Julian's position on mostly everything. She's a daddy's girl. That doesn't mean she doesn't adore you. It simply means she has great admiration for most everything concerning her father because she knows how much he adores her," she explained. "Are you both ready to answer all of her questions? She's been asking me so many things already, as if I'm totally in the loop on everything," Mom smiled even more as she stopped talking only to hear an immediate answer from me.

"Well, we're all going to dinner on Friday night. We both know that Emmy's ridiculously excited, although there's still quite a bit to figure out. Nevertheless, the toughest parts are already worked out. Julian and I's hearts are obviously in the right place personally, and with each other. We've both decided it would be totally wise and necessary to do some counseling together and as a family. Simply being in love with someone doesn't answer every question, and it doesn't conquer every challenge, past or present. Friday night will mostly be about us fully deciding and announcing what our next steps are as a family, and which roof we'll place our family under." I could feel my face smiling even more as I pondered upon everything I shared with Mom.

"So, you two are pretty much in love again? This isn't a slight rebound on either end?" Mom peered at me even closer to take in the response she obviously wanted.

"Yes, we're in love again. Julian and I have been through far too much both together and separately to take these next steps lightly or step into this haphazardly. And, with the way we know this will ultimately impact Emmy, we want to take every measure to do it well," I replied with the same confidence and comfort in my heart I'd sensed when I'd first told my parents about the awesome guy who I'd met at grad school. "I'm not terrified that he'll take an opportunity to cheat on me again, and he's not frightened that I'll stop taking care of myself or our marriage all over again."

"So... you guys are going to get married again?" Mom squealed with delight, tears immediately streaming down her face. "I'm so happy I could just scream, Whit."

"Thank you, Mom. And, you are practically screaming," I laughed out loud as I teased her. "But yes, we're getting hitched again. It would be a bit silly for us to be a strange version of boyfriend and girlfriend when we've already been married before, and our kid would obviously be more secure in all of it too. And no, we haven't set a date just yet or any other major details along those lines. We kind of want to fully decide which house we'll be living in first to keep Emmy stable in school and all of her activities," I smiled at her face that was still beaming with tear stains.

"That's perfectly okay. Wedding stuff is definitely steps that can be figured out as you guys are figuring out all of your other steps to be figured out." Mom grinned, attempting to hold in her next squeal.

"Speaking of next steps, Mom, you never got back to me on that training info for the cycling instructor program. I'm really serious about wanting to get that done." I beamed, realizing yet again how different life had become concerning my life.

"I actually emailed everything to you a couple of days ago. I can send it again to you, or we can just pull it up here on the laptop," Mom responded with complete glee in her voice. "I'm so excited you're going to be a fitness instructor."

"So am I. However, the moment I mentioned it to my personal trainer weeks ago, she took the news as full confirmation to kill me even more in our training sessions together. That's one of the main reasons I blasted through this past interval of weight loss results," I laughed as Mom grinned at me with a completely empathetic look. "I just realized one day during a deep conversation she and I had about why I'm committed to my fitness goals that I've always wanted to do something like this. Part of the reason I think I lived in annoyance at Barb and my colleague Kristina and so many other ladies who seemed to have it all together in their fitness journeys is because I so desperately wanted to not only be the woman who's in shape but also be that woman who's commitment and focus inspires and encourages someone else to get fit and healthy, and ultimately change their lives and stay on course with it."

"Whit, that's so awesome. How long have you been considering this?" Mom beamed.

"As long as I can remember actually, Mom. Honestly, as long as I've been using the nickname Little Miss Healthy Pants to describe every woman who I always thought was the best example of what I secretly longed to be," I continued speaking more openly and honestly than I had in years with my Mom. "Of course I'm not looking to change my career or anything. I love what I do in Dermatology. However, to be able to inspire a few women a couple of times a week like so many women have inspired me would be so awesome. It would be really awesome."

"It will be really awesome, and you'll be amazing at it, Whit. It's so much fun doing my classes as I know I'm helping people change their lives. And you definitely know both sides of the coin," she continued on as she affirmed my goals. "There you were feeling like you couldn't do anything to change your life. Then, you pushed forward through so much pain and disappointment to change your life in such a way that you're now a shining example to everyone around you. You're going to be so awesome at helping others help themselves, Whit."

"Thank you, Mom. I sure hope so." I beamed with gratitude at her positive words that seemed to place even more pep in my step for the days yet ahead.

"So, Dad, I was thinking. Since you're obviously not going to be marrying Miss Karen anymore, why don't we just go to Hawaii for Thanksgiving as a family? I'm sure you've probably already paid for the entire trip because I know you buy everything way sooner than you have to. Like, remember when I went into the hall closet that time and saw you had already bought my birthday gift right after Christmas although my birthday is in August?" Emily stared directly at Julian with a grin as he and I glanced at each other while trying our damnedest not to laugh at the brazenness of our child.

"Well, that's actually a pretty good idea for Thanksgiving, Emmy. Did your Mom put you up to suggesting that for us?" Julian winked at me, knowing the truth of his teasing response to her.

"Nope, I actually didn't even mention it to Mom because I knew she would try to talk me out of thinking about it, or even tell me not to bring it up to you. Probably because you guys are still playing ring around the rosy with completely getting back together," she laughed while searching our faces for any expression to confirm what she wanted to know before we began the process of telling here everything she needed to know. "What are you guys going to do anyway? I know that you're hanging out a lot together because I'm always at Grandma's now. Dad, you broke up with Karen months ago, and Mom, you lost Cory a long time ago. I'm not saying I'm happy about any of that. Well, some of it I am," she smirked at Julian before we smirked at each other in acknowledgement of the funny she made.

"Well, that's what we actually came out tonight as a family for, Emmy. We're here to discuss the future of our family. So, you're asking what are we're going to do," Julian smiled at her with so much love in his voice and eyes. "We're going to bring our family back together. Mom and I love each other deeply, and we want to continue raising you to be an amazing young lady. We want our family together with the love we have for one another."

"So you're saying that I'm not going to have to live at one house during the week and another house on the weekends anymore," she beamed as she literally bounced up and down in her chair. "Wait, but now there's going to be even more of the same healthy, crazy food in the fridge and the pantry?"

"Yes, young lady. We'll still have lots of veggies and healthy snacks. And, we'll have chips without a normal name on the bag," I chuckled at her typical pre-teen response. "The main thing we want to discuss with you though is which house we'll be living in for now until we ultimately sell both houses and buy or build an entirely different family home."

"We're going to get a new house? Is it going to be with stuff that I actually like inside of it?" She gave us both an exasperated look, as if she paid every bill at home. "Will it have a really great pool like Uncle Rick and Aunt Barb's, or will it be an old school one like the one at Dad's."

"Old school?" Julian and I laughed out loud simultaneously at our way too grown up little girl.

"Yes, old school," Emily shot back as she laughed even harder. "Like, no longer cool but maybe cool when you were both in school a long, long time ago."

"Uh, we are still cool, young lady," Julian replied as he shuffled at his tie and shot his signature smirk at her. "Well, at least your dad's cool quotient isn't going anywhere. We're still working on getting Mom in to retest for her cool badge."

"Ha-ha! Just the fact that you called it a cool badge proves you are not cool," I laughed out loud again at how hilarious Julian could be just at being himself. "You're handsome, and you're still mostly hot. But, you're not cool, my love."

"Mostly hot? I am hot." Julian responded with a fake snarl as he pretended to be crushed by my teasing comment. "If you weren't so gorgeous, my hotness would totally outshine all of that. I'll deal with it though because I like you being gorgeous, babe."

"Ugh, enough with the pet names, out loud," Emily interrupted our blissful bantering back and forth with a comical look of disgust. "Next you'll be kissing, out loud. And let's not forget, you're in public with your kid."

"Well now that you've mentioned it, Emmy, I didn't get a proper kiss from Mom earlier." Julian retorted, looking directly at me before using the most disgustingly embarrassing sexy tone he could find to distort his deep voice to tease Emily while I laughed uncontrollably. "Sweetheart, we must lock our lips in unbridled love at this very moment."

"You're absolutely right, my hot, hunky, handsome lover boy," I giggled, joining in on the mortification of our adorable daughter. "Bring those lips across this round table and make me spin with even more ove and devotion," I grinned as Julian reached over to kiss me in a far more sweet than silly manner.

"Ugh, Mom! Aren't we supposed to be talking about which house we're all going to live in?" Emily giggled and gagged simultaneously. her olive skin turning fairly crimson at our behavior. "Shouldn't you guys wait to get home and completely inside of the house to do all of your ooey gooey cooing and kissing?"

"Oh, yes. We were talking about where to live before you, my sweet child, changed the subject about how we don't know how to be cool. So, you deserved that one," I laughed a bit more before responding to her. "But yes, we've made a decision, and we know you'll be pretty happy about it. Dad's going to move in with us, and we'll sell the house he's in now before we begin looking for or building another one. Dad's house has a lot of old memories of the family we used to be, so it'll be great to temporarily get going again where you and I are before we move to a new home and build completely new memories together. Even more importantly, you won't have to change schools. What do you think?" I finished.

"That's fine because neither of the two houses have ever felt like home to me," she smiled, responding in her signature honesty mode. "I've always just felt like I'm just visiting both places. Just a longer visit at Mom's than at yours, Dad. It's not like they're not good houses. It just doesn't feel like home when one parent just told you 'Bye' a couple of days before and the other parent already has to start counting down the days to tell you 'Bye' again."

"Well, we had no idea you felt that way, Emmy. We had no idea," I responded with a brief surge of guilt for what she'd experienced over the past few years due to our choices. "I guess it's even better that we'll all be together as a family again."

"Yeah, divorce sucks. I know a lot of parents do it now, whether they have to or not, but it sucks," she responded like a completely sufficient grownup yet totally dependent child again. "Although I'm kind of scared it could always happen again, I'm happy you guys are going to try to be together again. I'm really happy."

"Well, I'm very happy that you're happy, baby girl, because we surely are. And, I don't want you scared about anything," Julian replied while Emily and I both beamed at the man we adored. "It means the world to me to have both of my girls back in my life again. Although I can't change anything about the past, I am going to make sure the future is so much better for all of us. I know that I've said it before to both of you ladies, but I apologize for what I did to hurt our family before. I'm sorry I violated your complete trust in me, Whitty. Emmy, I'm sorry I showed you that your dad couldn't be totally reliable by cheating on your mom. Although I'll never be a perfect man, you both can certainly trust me when I say I'll always be faithful to Mom, and show you and her that I can be trusted to protect your heart from experiencing any kind of betrayal or abandonment because of my behavior. I love you ladies, and I'm so grateful to have you back in my life," he finished with what I was sure was tears glistening in his brown eyes.

"See! That's why we have to go to Hawaii for Thanksgiving, Dad! That's the type of stuff you can say to Mom in Hawaii! You can say it all over again on the beach," Emily squealed as she took in the magnitude of what Julian had conveyed to her and I. "Take her there and say that stuff to her, Dad. And, you can marry her again over there. You guys are getting married again, right? Just do it in Hawaii. I'll even say yes this time to staying there the entire 10 days," she laughed.

"Ha-ha! Are you really only 12 years old, child? I think the doctors made an error on your birth certificate." I laughed in enthusiasm and slight embarrassment of all she had said. "Yes, Dad and I are getting married again, but what you're trying to plan would be only weeks away. Even more, I honestly wouldn't want to get married on a second hand version of a trip that was already planned. We've already talked about getting married, and we'll definitely do so soon, but it'll be even better than Hawaii."

"What's better than getting married in Hawaii, Mom?" Emily threw up her arms in her hilarious drama queen mode.

"Mom's absolutely right." Julian responded to her. "There's too many gorgeous places in the world for us to re-marry on a do-over trip. But, I'm sure we can definitely take that paid for trip to Hawaii for Thanksgiving as a family. That's if Mom and I can work out both our schedules for it," he smiled at me for a nod of approval.

"I'm sure I can somehow take the time off. My cycling instructor certification is the week after Thanksgiving. If they hire me on the schedule to teach classes at Mom's facility, I'll begin instructing only a couple of weeks after that." I thought more out loud to myself than just in response to Julian.

"Well, we certainly don't want to interrupt your fitness aspirations, Little Miss Healthy Pants, but we can find a way to work around it." He laughed as he blew a sweet kiss at me across the table.

"Ha-ha! I can't believe you're using my formerly foul name against me, but I'll take it. And, I'll take that trip with you," I giggled back at him as my heart fluttered with the joy it felt in being in love all over again with the man who I had never quite closed my heart to. "We'll all take it, and we'll get it all worked out. I've got lots of vacation time that I didn't really use this past summer with everything that went on. In fact, the med spa has actually been expecting me to take a sabbatical ever since then. I didn't even celebrate my birthday in July."

"Well, let's do it, my love. Let's also make sure you pack nothing but swimsuits for the trip," he grinned as we both knew that Emily would be embarrassed yet again by our chit-chat.

"I will definitely do so, handsome. Can't wait to snorkel hand in hand with you." I beamed back.

"You guys! Really?" Emily rolled her eyes with a smirk. "They're bringing out our food now!"

"Emmy, you would not be sitting here mortified at us if we hadn't had conversations like this 12 years ago." I laughed as I shot back at her.

"And, even before then." Julian added with an even louder laugh.

"Please spare me the details before I take back all of my happiness of being so happy for the both of you right now." Emily laughed, beaming at Julian and me with full approval in her brown eyes of the new plans for our new version of family again.

"Have I already told you how ridiculously happy I am for you?" Barb grinned at me as we continued to shuffle around for a few moments in absolute bliss before class began.

"Yes, almost 100 times today alone. And each time makes me more and more nervous," I chuckled, thinking about the hour ahead of me and the year behind me simultaneously.

Our family trip to Hawaii had been full of huge surprises and sappy festivities of love as Julian had officially proposed to me under a gorgeous sunset with our darling Emily beaming on in full cahoots of it all. Although every box wasn't unpacked, nor was every piece of furniture decided upon of what to keep or toss, we were all under one roof again. No matter how exhausting the day was before we arrived home or how late the nights were getting ready for the next day ahead, it felt amazing to wake up to all of it with Julian and to crash comfortably in his arms afterwards.

"I don't mean to make you nervous, Whit. It just makes me so happy to see you so happy. And, with Julian, mind you," she giggled at me. "Now, you're in a position where you're going to be instructing and inspiring other people. What the hell!" She finished with a wide grin and a squeal.

I'd breezed through my cycling instructor certification training weeks ago as the additional 10-12 pounds I'd dropped in my final phase of training with Sabrina immensely increased my cardio endurance and confidence. I was 136 pounds of lean muscle and full energy. Although I knew I looked better than I ever had as I pranced around in a size 4, I felt even better. Here I was I mentally prepared to help other individuals do what I had once never imagined having the courage or willpower to do myself.

"I know. Little Miss Healthy Pants has a lot to be thankful for." I responded, making us both laugh incredibly hard while finishing the setup of our bikes in the studio before I continued to wait anxiously with ease to instruct my first cycling class. "Thank you so much for being here with me. It means so much to me, Barb."

"You know I wouldn't miss this for the world, Whit. You're my sister," she grinned. "You're the craziest version of one I could ever have, but you're still mine."

"And, I think those ladies coming in are all mine." I beamed as the first few women walked into the studio to choose their bike.

"They are, and so am I." Barb squealed. "You'd better bring it, Whit."

"You'd better park it so I can bring it, girlfriend." I giggled at her as I looked over to greet the ladies.

"Oh, I'm going to right now," Barb snickered as she walked away to hop on her bike.

"Good morning ladies. Welcome to Cycle Blast. I'm your instructor today, Whitney Cordona. Feel free to call me Whit."

Acknowledgements

I am so grateful for the many amazing friends and family members who frame my life with love and support far beyond the writing process. Although I'd like to personally thank each and every one of you 'on paper', I do think it's best that the content of the chapters of my first book be just a bit larger than my listing of acknowledgements. <Insert huge laugh and huge hug to all of you, written and unwritten>

Daddy, your wisdom, hilarity, and support infuses my soul with confidence through every tear and triumph. I adore you too, and I'm happy to now admit that you told me so.

Mommy, your love for me has always been filled with so much admiration and hopefulness. Thank you for always giving me the best of you. My love for you is as huge as your contagious laugh.

Catera, you were the first set of creative eyes to confirm this wasn't a project to continue to put off. If I could chat with my 17 year old self, I'd tell her everything she's experiencing is to be able to one day tell her amazing niece that 17 and beyond is as wonderful as she chooses to make it. I love you.

Wes, your encouragement and insight has always been relentless in challenging me to be the individual I was clearly created to be. Thank you for being such a great friend and the best ex-boyfriend a girl could ever have.

To my hardworking and hilarious family of Rockstars at Winspire— the fun, friendship, and family bond we've created is such a strength to my life. I love each of you far more than you love the words 'cooldown' and 'recover'.

To my friends and family at LifeTime Fitness— the courage to fully create this work was birth from the core of the years of good laughs and hard work I shared with so many of you. Thank you for teaching me that the only way to enjoy the bumpy ride of fitness is to make it a lifestyle.

To my entire "Blind Side" Cajun family, led by my dears Elman and Tina Authement— this endeavor is as much your celebration as it is mine. Thank you all for loving and believing in me long before I truly knew the gifts and treasures within me.

To my Fab Four BFF's: Belinda George, Felicia Lugo, Massie Bergeron, and Zoe Reyes— "Thank you for being a friend... Travel down the road and back again... Your heart is true... You're a pal and a confidant... And if you threw a party..." Ha-ha! Yes, I went there, and I'll continue to croon it until we're all completely golden. I love you ladies, and I thank you for embracing and encouraging the essence of how I tend to do this life stuff—happy, healthy, and to the beat of varied drums.

To my two little brothers, Cale McMellon and Chase Austin— thank you for being a double blessing of a void I never thought would be filled in my heart again. You two crazies are the best brothers I could've ever imagined.

And last but not least, there are a few specific individuals who've been nothing short of fabulous in the encouragement and support they've shown specifically during the process of my penning this first book.

Courtney Rhodes— thank you for challenging me, with passion and compassion, to take this book and the gifts on the inside of me completely off the shelf. Your insight, encouragement, and methodology is second to none. You are the mentor I aspire to be!

Rachelle Dungan and Sherrayne Martin— from my blogging to this book, your encouragement to continue on in every sentence that's come out of my soul has been so many fresh winds of inspiration to me. The book is written and many more to come!

Brandi Neal and Donna Guidry— your words of enthusiasm have been strength to my soul, not only because of your thoughtful support but also because of the sincerity of your heart in every facet of it. I love and admire you too!

Joni Claville and Deborah Jones— thank you for speaking and listening in ways that have always reminded me that the spirit of who and what I am matters far beyond anything I do or don't feel. Our sisterhood is a Godsend!

May you all enjoy the gift of the creativity you've encouraged and supported. I love you!

Q & A with author
SONIA MARIE TRIMBLE

Who is this Sonia Marie Trimble?

I'm a fun loving, fitness driven woman who's seriously, incredibly, ridiculously excited to become 40 years of age this summer. Seriously. I feel as though I'm finally growing up and growing awake to all life entails for me, and I'm no longer afraid to live fully. I'm honored to serve and impact individuals in my fitness career. I'm grateful for the guidance and grace of God in my life. And I'm in love with my amazing friends and family who lovingly surround me with support through the craziness of all my craziness.

Have you always wanted to be a writer?

As a young adult, I wrote poetry, songs, and short stories. I've always recognized that there's a gift of writing on the inside of me. However, it took years of maturity to occur in me before I decided to start truly cultivating my gift, knowing that sharing my work isn't about attempting to create material which I hope everyone applauds and approves of. I'm finding that good writing is about being authentic to my own voice as I write with complete freedom, bringing forth my own personal insight and energy to connect with those who are yearning to read and hear the words I've penned.

How does it feel to have written your first novel?

It feels absolutely amazing to see this dream, which I had shelved for almost two years, alive and in print.

What suggestion(s) as a new writer do you have for other aspiring writers?

Please give attention to the ideas that are ruminating inside of you. Many works of art, especially in writing, we deem amazing today began with a simple idea that was almost ignored. Also, try to read far more than you write. While no specific book sparked my initial idea of this book, reading books have always breathed life and fresh energy into me, especially during my own writing process.

What did you enjoy most about writing Fit Happens?

I really enjoyed writing the conversations between Whitney and the other characters. There are specific times I can recall giggling or even becoming teary eyed at my laptop as the words poured from my soul, through my fingers, and unto the page. Two of my favorite dialogues are the heart to heart she had with Olivia in Chapter 2, and the exchange between her and Cory in Chapter 7.

What did you enjoy least about the writing process?

Going through the multiple drafts of making Whitney's story what I knew it needed to be was unbelievably tough. While it's exhilarating to pen those initial words of each chapter, it can become exhausting to go back to the manuscript to expound just a bit more, or remove something or someone which no longer works for the big picture of the work at hand. Chapter 2 was my toughest in working through this process, but I found it was always worth every tough moment.

Where did you get the name "Little Miss Healthy Pants"?

Growing up in the south, the ability to express sugary sweet sarcasm flows as freely as iced tea in the summer. The term just fit, as I knew I wanted Whitney's voice to convey an air of hilarious mockery as she attempted to mask the pain and insecurities that hindered her.

Why did you choose Dallas, Texas as the setting of your novel?

I lived in Dallas with my dad for a while as a teenager. Although I didn't decide to make it my official home as an adult, I always enjoy my time there when I go to visit family and friends. Dallas is no doubt a gem of the south, with the dynamism and perks of most anything included in a great metropolitan city.

Who are your favorite characters in the book?

That's such a tough question. I loved everyone, except maybe Karen. <insert laughter and applause> I had an amazing time pulling for Whitney through the highs and lows of her journey, and I certainly relate to the temperament and thought process of Sabrina. However, Barb and Olivia are my absolute favorites. Barb is a refreshing portrayal of a woman who's as beautiful on the inside as she is outwardly, and her consistent behavior towards Whitney is a great reminder of the value of good friendship in our lives. Olivia simply rocks. She is the mentor or wise big sister we're either blessed with in our lives, or we spend a lifetime longing to have someone like her. Her spunk and hilarity was so much fun to pen, and it made my heart smile to see the strength and support she showered upon Whitney.

What's next for Little Miss Healthy Pants?

The courage to complete Fit Happens gave me such clarity for the next steps. Fit Happens is one of five books in the companion series of Little Miss Healthy Pants. Though Whitney was the star of Fit Happens, the next books will feature various characters from her story as the main. Book 2 will feature her daughter Emily, in Emily's voice. We'll meet Emily as a 16-year-old junior in high school facing the challenges of body image and bullying that far too many young adults face today. However, she'll face her fears and her frenemies [worst enemy with a best friend persona] with a confidence that will speak hope and empowerment to our beautiful teens, twentysomethings, and the parents of such. Emily will inspire us all to tap into our inner brave girl, remembering that no matter who's in our face or who's at our side, we are only as amazing and as beautiful as we choose to be.

www.littlemisshealthypants.com

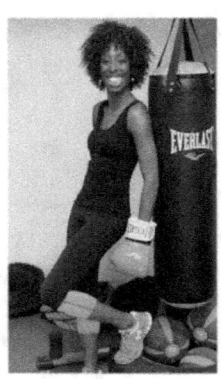

ABOUT THE AUTHOR

Sonia Marie Trimble is a NASM certified personal trainer who's been in the health and fitness industry for seven years. When she isn't writing, Sonia can be found training with her amazing clients at her fitness studio in Houma, Louisiana. She chronicles their hilarious and hardworking sessions on Facebook and Instagram.

Fit Happens is her first novel. A companion of it, "Little Miss Healthy Pants $E = mc^{3"}$, yes cubed, is currently in the works.

www.littlemisshealthypants.com

Connect with the Author:
Facebook: @littlemisshealthypantsbook
Instagram: @littlemisshealthypants
Twitter: @littlemissSMT